Understanding and treating trauma-related dissociation

in CPTSD (complex PTSD) and DID (Dissociative Identity Disorder) following exposure to sexual abuse as a child

Me nobody owns

Understanding and treating trauma-related dissociation

in CPTSD (complex PTSD) and DID (Dissociative Identity Disorder) following exposure to sexual abuse as a child

By Maja Koppfeldt
Licensed Psychotherapist, Sexologist

Max Winston
PUBLISHING

Understanding and treating trauma-related dissociation

First edition

ISBN 978-91-989289-3-8

Cover and graphic design:	Vestergård webb & design (www.vestergard.se)
Print:	Libri Plureos GmbH, Friedensallee 273, 22763 Hamburg, Germany
Publishers:	Max Winston Publishing

Table of contents

Preface **11**

Prevalence **13**

WONSA *15*

Recommendations *17*

ACE (Adverse Childhood Experiences) *19*

SAIS (Sexual Abuse Injury Syndrome) *19*

Incest **23**

A confused dynamic *28*

Connection *31*

Possible motives for incest *33*

Resistance always exists *35*

Incest in culture *36*

Child sexual abuse material **39**

AI identifies vulnerable children *41*

Detecting sexual abuse of young children **43**

Physical signs of child sexual abuse *43*

The Disclosure - Receiving a Story *49*

How sexual abuse affects health as an adult **55**

Treatment SAIS, 1-4 PTSD and CPTSD **61**

Transference and countertransference *63*

Subjective perspective *65*

A safe place *66*

Villa Solviken *67*

The relationship to anger 72
Tolerance window 73
Resilience 73
Forgiveness 74
Spirituality 75
Organization, work environment and self-care 76
Lifespan Integration 77
Group therapy 78
Documentation 79
Active defenses in survivors 81
Denial 82
Primitive withdrawal 83
Projecting 84
Turning towards the self 85
Sexualisation 86
Sex for money 87
Sex as self-harm 88
Sublimation 90
Splitting of the self 94
Dissociation 95
Division 96
Dissociation in the body 97
Amnesia 99
A first fragmentation 101
What affects the degree of dissociation? 103
How long you have been exposed 103
How frequent the abuse has been 105
Penetrating assault 106
Degree of violence, coercion and intimidation 107
A male perpetrator 109

The closeness of the relationship ... 109
Passive or willing participation ... 111
Involuntary erotic response ... 112
Guilt, shame, disgust ... 114
The Westermarck effect - feeling of disgust ... 116
Betrayal, horror and confusion ... 119
Fight, Flight ... 120
– Freeze ... 121
– Fawn ... 122
Gang rapes ... 123
DID (Dissociative Identity Disorder) ... **125**
Three phase therapy ... 129
Cultural perspectives on DID ... 131
– Western Perspectives: Psychological Fragmentation in North America and Europe ... 132
– South Asia: Possessed parts and spiritual narratives ... 133
– East Asia: Somatic and masked presentations ... 133
– Africa: Ancestral Spirits and Social Acceptance ... 134
– Latin America: Syncretic Faith and Emotional Outbursts ... 134
Skepticism towards DID ... 135
DID in culture ... 136
Neurological insights into DID ... **139**
– Structural Changes: Trauma's Lasting Imprint on the Brain ... 140
– Functional Dynamics: The Neural Dance of Identity Shifts ... 140
– Clinical implications: A bridge between research and practice ... 141
– Conclusions ... 142
Parts ... **143**
Fawn or Feign parts ... 146
Perpetrator parts ... 147
Somatoform Dissociation ... 150

Constructed DID **153**
Mind Control *153*
Programming *156*
Strategies perpetrators use to achieve sub-ego *158*
– Conditioning- operant, classical, fear conditioning *158*
– Fear conditioning *159*
– Fraud *160*
– Hypnosis *161*
– Forced abuse *161*
– Identification with aggressor *162*
– Deprivation of basic needs *164*
– Direct terrorization *164*
– Indoctrination into the perpetrators' beliefs or agenda *164*
Protracted abuse *165*
Organized and ritual sexual abuse of children **171**
Pedophiles **177**
Pedophile manual *179*
Female perpetrators *181*
Misogynistic attitudes *185*
Treatment SAIS, 5-6 CPTSD and DID **187**
Talking through *187*
The Trauma curve by Dr. Eric Wolterstroff *188*
Top of mind model SAIS 5-6 .... **191**
Phase 1: Initial stabilization and mapping *194*
Phase 2 The trauma treatment *200*
Phase 3: Final phase *206*
AI as a tool *207*
MDMA assisted therapy - the future of trauma treatment *209*
Final words *210*
References **213**

About the author 232

Preface

The book highlights, among other things, the damage that sexual abuse of a child generates, not only acute damage in childhood but also the damage that the patient carries with him throughout his life. The book follows a common thread and goes from milder sexual abuse of children to extreme, torture-like sexual abuse of children with organized and ritual elements. The book describes treatment methods and how the treatment needs to be adapted to the damage that the patient has suffered through the sexual abuse. The book links the patient's damage to the degree of sexual abuse they were subjected to as a child and in adulthood and with a special focus on the diagnosis DID (Dissociative identity disorder) previously called Multiple personality disorder (MP), an often incorrectly presented illness, where the diagnostic applications are used inadequately and the illness has been sensationalized to some extent. It is not possible to understand or treat DID without also acknowledging the terrifying fact of how children are sexually exploited, exposed to extreme terror or neglected. The majority of people diagnosed with DID have survived early, repeated and prolonged extreme sexual abuse as children. A person with DID experiences shifts in their identity and between different personalities, each identity can take control of behaviors at different times and has a distinct pattern of thoughts and how they relate to the world. Amnesia occurs when one part may be completely unaware of what is happening when another part is prominent. DID can be overlooked both for its polysymptomatic profile and the tendency of patients to feel shame and thus avoid showing the dissociative symptoms and telling about their history of sexual abuse as a child. If the disease is not recognized by clinicians, professionals cannot provide the patient with the right treatment based on the guidelines that exist. The cost of ignoring DID as a diagnosis is high, not only for the affected patients but for the entire support system such as their family and friends, the health care system and society as a whole (Brand et al., 2016). DID is a complex trauma-related diagnosis characterized by 2 or more distinct identity stages and recurrent amnesia. The diagnosis often arises after severe childhood abuse, such as sexual abuse. With a prevalence of 1.1-1.5% in the general population, which can be compared to schizophrenia, DID is a significant health and medical issue. Despite this, DID is a diagnosis that is rarely diagnosed in Sweden. DID is underdiagnosed due to a lack of clinical attention and stubborn skepticism. Most people recoil and do not want to listen when sexual abuse of children is mentioned. Many doubt the accuracy of the information, but even when people want to listen, they cannot grasp the magnitude, they simply cannot believe that such things happen in our civilized part of the world. Perpetrators in turn exploit this belief when they tell their victims that no one will believe you. Not believing in statistics about the prevalence of child sexual abuse in our society can be likened to not believing in gang crime. It exists even if we don't see it. We know that those of us who have grown up in safety and security have sometimes accepted the myth that there are no people who exploit and torture children in organized contexts in civilized Western society. Therapists know how difficult it is for survivors to talk about horrific truths and memories, although, unfortunately, not many therapists have the capacity or the patience to listen to this level of child sexual abuse. The book describes the Top of Mind model, which was developed specifically to be able to treat trauma-related dissociation after sexual abuse based on different degrees of severity. The Top of Mind model is an eclectic method aimed at clinicians who wish to deepen their knowledge of trauma and dissociative symptoms for patients after sexual abuse. I have spent a large part of my life as a clinician trying to understand, at times it has required everything from me to be able to grasp the extent of the crime my patients were subjected to, its consequences and driving forces. I believe that people who have experienced terrible abuse in childhood can, with courage and strength, find the truth about what happened to them as children and through treatment achieve a safe and healthy life in the present.

As a society, we need to research, pay attention to and discuss sexual abuse against children continuously in order to develop social services, the legal system, laws, health care, change outdated views, educate and modify our perceptions based on what reality actually looks like. Otherwise, we risk relativizing sexual violence against children. The visibility of sexual abuse needs to be highlighted in order to make otherwise private structures a collective concern.

Prevalence

It is more common for people with experience of sexual trauma to be in healthcare than for the normal population Young-Wolff, (2018); referenced in Wiman, (2022). WHO (World Health Organization) has examined broader definitions of violence and sexual violence and shows that approximately 20–35% of all women have such experiences. In incest, the victims are 80% women and 20% men and according to WHO, 96% of incestuous abuse is carried out by men. Several studies indicate that approximately 28% of women and 10% of men in the general population have experienced sexual abuse before the age of 14 (Loeb et al., 2002). A general meaning of sexual abuse against children includes both abuse in the form of physical contact where the perpetrator touches the child sexually, forcing the child to touching themselves. Or the perpetrator through oral, anal or vaginal sex, through acts that do not involve physical contact between the child and the perpetrator, such as exposing oneself, the child being asked to take pictures/film on themselves (Ekdahl, 2017). Of the children living in Sweden today, it is estimated that one in five children have been subjected to sexual abuse (Landberg et al. 2015). Of these, less than 10% come to the attention of social services or the police. International studies show similar figures. According to figures from the Swedish Council for Crime Prevention (Brå), children aged 0–17 are three times more likely to be raped than an adult. Girls aged 15–17 are more than 6 times more likely to be raped than an adult. More recent research suggests that incest between siblings, primarily between an older brother and a younger sister, is the most common form of incest Carlson, Maciol & Schneider, (2006); referenced in McGuian & Stephenson, (2014).

Estimating the prevalence of incest is difficult due to a high risk of memory bias that is part of the nature of incest. As well as the high dropout rates of respondents due to fear of survivor shame, a fear of being socially labeled, ridiculed, despised, distrusted and alienated Sariola & Uutela, (1996); referenced in Shaked, Bensimon & Mashiack, (2021). Incest victims in general, rarely receive recognition or understanding from either society or the legal system (Schulz, 2014). According to Statistics Sweden (2013), there are approximately 940,000 girls aged 0–17 years in Sweden and according to Svedin and Banch's (2002) report, six to seven percent of all girls have been exposed to incest one or more times during their lifetime. This means that between 55–65,000 girls in Sweden were exposed to incest (2013). Reports are increasing annually and this is probably correlated to increased awareness in society, but the hidden number is still large (Frank, 2003). The hidden number refers to the number of undetected or unreported abuses. Landberg et al; (2015); referenced in Johansson & Svedin, (2021) found that approximately one in five 18-year-olds has been exposed to some form of sexual abuse during their childhood (approximately one in ten boys and one in three girls). In Sweden, around 19,000 sexual crimes are reported to the police each year, but many refrain from reporting them and the number of convictions is misleading if we want to understand how common sexual crime is (Brå). Berliner and Elliott (2002) believe that since childhood sexual abuse is underreported, prevalence is best measured in retrospective studies with adult respondents.

According to Foote and Park, (2008); referenced in Howell (2011) there is sufficient data in the world to show that DID is no rarer than schizophrenia. One possible explanation for the perception that DID is rare is due to the public belief that child sexual abuse is rare. There is a myth that DID is an overdiagnosed condition and primarily a phenomenon that originated in North America and was only diagnosed by DID specialists (Paris; referenced in Brandt et al., 2016). However, the empirical literature indicates that diagnosed DID patients are found all over the world and that the clinicians who diagnose patients with DID have different training and experience with DID. According to Brandt, et al., (2016), DID is considered to be underdiagnosed rather than overdiagnosed. Studies show that most individuals diagnosed with DID have been in the healthcare system for 6-12 years before they are correctly diagnosed with DID. Studies from Australia, China and Turkey have found that DID patients are often misdiagnosed. There are several different studies that point to different figures for the prevalence of DID in the population, Brandt et al., (2016) believe that DID is found in 1.1%-1.5% of the population. Similar studies conducted in Turkey show that 1.1% of women (n= 628) have DID. According to DSM-5, the 12-month prevalence of DID is estimated to be 1.5% of the adult American population (American Psychiatric Association 2013). The prevalence in psychiatry has been estimated to be about 5% (variation from 0.4%-14%), (Sar, 2011; referenced in Huntjens et al., 2018).

WONSA

Wonsa (World Of No Sexual Abuse) was founded in 2014 by Gita Rajan, a general practitioner and specialist in general medicine, and for 10 years was Sweden's only specialist clinic for victims of sexual violence in a non-acute stage. Wonsa has a vision of a world free from sexual abuse. By working with research, treatment and education, the foundation developed and disseminated initiatives that prevent sexual abuse. Wonsa currently runs a training platform where healthcare professionals who meet the target group of victims of sexual violence can train and certify themselves based on the SAIS (Sexually Abused Injury Syndrome) degree of traumatization. Sexual abuse and sexual violence are areas characterized by aggression, the exercise of power, taboo, shame, guilt, politics and opinions. Wonsa is convinced that in order to constructively navigate through this minefield, knowledge, courage and empathy are required. Between 2014 and 2025, the Wonsa Foundation has operated specialized clinics for the treatment of post-traumatic stress disorder (PTSD), complex PTSD (CPTSD) and dissociative identity disorder (DID) after sexual assault. The distribution between PTSD, CPTSD and DID has been 10/70/20 since the start. The patients have had a high degree of comorbidity, with an average of six diagnoses at the time of first contact with Wonsa. The majority of patients have sought help from other healthcare providers before coming to Wonsa and over 30% of patients have attempted suicide at least once before starting their treatment at Wonsa. The average treatment time for a patient with simple PTSD is 4.4 treatments. For patients with severe PTSD or mild CPTSD, the treatment time has been between 6 months and 2 years. The average treatment time for a patient with more severe CPTSD or DID, often after long-term incest, trafficking and/or ritual abuse from early childhood, is 3-5 years and 8-10 years respectively. The treatment time may seem long, but it is important to consider that these patients have often been in psychiatry for many years, not infrequently for decades. It has often been assessed as therapy *refractory* (a condition that is resistant or refractory to treatment) or *not treatable before* they arrived in Wonsa.

Method development to help CPTSD and DID patients with shorter treatment times has been a priority area within Wonsa. Among patients with CPTSD and DID, Wonsa's experience is that the total burden of illness, including both somatic and psychiatric comorbidity, as well as suicidality, increases with the proportion of ACEs (Adverse Childhood Experiences) that a patient has. Many have spent decades in regionally run psychiatric services before coming to Wonsa. They have often received several different diagnoses with respective treatments, including medications for psychosis and bipolar disorder. They often have long sick leave periods (several years) and it is common for the patients to be on addictive medications. For patients with CPTSD and DID, the primary goal of treatment, as for patients with PTSD, is for the patients' injuries to heal and for the patients to become symptom-free and able to work.

Wonsa's experience with these patients is that they consist of four main groups: Patients with DID and CDID (Complex DID), patients with severe (CPTSD+) and mild dissociation (CPTSD). Wonsa's experience is that patients with severe dissociative states in particular need long treatment periods with parallel interventions that include methods and medications that are not (yet) within the framework of the treatment programs and national guidelines that currently exist in Sweden for PTSD.

According to Wonsa, there is some evidence that intensive psychotherapy with multiple interventions, as well as with psychedelics, can shorten the treatment time significantly. Wonsa's experience shows that some patients with CPTSD and DID who have gone a long time without adequate treatment and where the opportunity for inpatient intensive psychotherapy or treatment with psychedelics has not been given, have incurred permanent disabilities. For these, the goal is symptom relief, lasting sickness compensation and the opportunity for a meaningful life.

Based on this, Wonsa sees that the following quality indicators may be appropriate when evaluating treatment for patients with CPTSD and DID:

Proportion screened for ACEs and investigate type of sexual violence exposure
Number of patients who have healed injuries/have completed treatment and are starting to return to work
Number of patients who are "non-responders" (patients who do not respond to given treatment) and "drop-outs" (patients who choose to discontinue treatment).
Percentage of non-responders and drop-outs where underlying cause has been analyzed
Number of patients receiving sickness compensation
Percentage of patients who experience improved quality of life after sickness compensation
Number who have had addictive drugs introduced, tapered or discontinued
Number of serious suicide attempts or completed suicides

Recommendations

Wonsa's recommendations for continued care development are based on experience from 10 years of work with the patient group, international literature and feedback from patients.

Use ICD 11 to avoid confusing the diagnosis of CPTSD with the DSM 5 diagnosis PTSD with dissociative subtype, which is a more severe form of PTSD, for which there is treatment programs and guidelines.
Screen all patients for ACEs and type of sexual violence exposure. This helps to understand the degree of injury underlying the widespread symptoms that often occur.

Discriminate between CPTDS/CPTSD+ and DID/CDID and thus facilitate treatment planning. It also provides a basis for objective analysis and structured improvement work regarding patients who do not respond to ("non-responders"), or choose to discontinue treatments ("drop-outs").
Follow up and analyze patients who discontinue or do not respond to treatments, and include them in the results.
Individualize treatment time, intensity, and methods, and don't be afraid to provide several different interventions in parallel or one after the other, timed based on the healing process and needs. For example, the nervous system may need to be calmed so that cognitive abilities are available, before CBT treatment begins. Another example is intensive psychotherapy, where exposure in the morning can be followed by integrated methods in the afternoon.
Use a less hierarchical structure between caregivers and patients, where dialogue and shared learning between caregivers and patients are encouraged. Wonsa's experience is that this increases participation, but above all increases a sense of context and meaning for the patients and reduces suicidality.
Dare to use off-label prescribing and avoid political bias in drug selection.

Wonsa is today an educational institute with a vision of a world in peace and tranquility. Wonsa's mission is to work to end sexual abuse in all its forms. They achieve their goals through knowledge, experience, factual observations, insights and integrity that they have built up and are constantly developing together with their colleagues and patients. Through courage, they create opportunities and break new ground when needed. But above all, they provide care, they never forget where Wonsa comes from and they understand that what is done or not done affects others.

ACE (Adverse Childhood Experiences)

ACE studies included nearly 18,000 people and identified what are now known as the ten strongest risk factors for early death and the development of mental and physical ill health in adulthood. ACE is one of the world's most cited public health studies and was conducted in the USA. It addresses how adverse or traumatic childhood experiences affect you as an adult. Seven categories examine childhood experiences in relation to ill health; psychological, physical, sexual abuse, violence against the mother, living/growing up with drug addicts, mental illness or suicide, if the parents have been in prison. The results show that the more ACEs a person has been exposed to, the greater the likelihood of more health risks later in life. According to the study, people with several ACEs in their luggage are at greater risk of having problems with alcohol, drugs, unemployment, smoking, lack of exercise and in addition to that they have an increased risk of obesity, diabetes, cancer, cardiovascular disease, stroke, depression and suicide attempts. It is usually said that the more ACEs, the greater the risk. In the worst case, life expectancy can be shortened by up to 20 years. Hanna Rundell, who researches ACEs in relation to public health, believes that there are great benefits to looking at parents and parenting from a holistic perspective and that even small challenges in parenting can look different if we have several ACEs in our luggage. But above all, we now have better knowledge about how we can prevent and counteract the harmful effects of adverse childhood experiences. Dr. Nadine Burk Harris gives a simple explanation of the ACE study in her 15-minute TED talk *How childhood trauma affects health across a lifetime.*

SAIS (Sexual Abuse Injury Syndrome)

The SAIS model was developed by Wonsa to grade sexual trauma. Sexual assault often brings trauma-related experiences such as fear, guilt, shame, betrayal and confusion to a head, because the intensity of these experiences was so strong when the memory was encoded. In retrospect, the memories become difficult to survive and live with. In order to survive and live with what happened, it is common for the experience of the event to be divided or fragmented. When the location of the event is one's own body, the experience of it is often also fragmented, which in turn risks creating mixed and deep dissociative states that make treatment difficult.

Just like *the risk* for what type of physical damage the body *can be expected* is affected by whether a person was exposed to low- or high-energy violence, for example what speed a car was driving at the time of the crash, Wonsa's experiences are based on *the risk* for the degree of fragmentation and neurobiological damage that can *be expected*, is influenced by the type of sexual violence experienced. It is important to understand that *risk and expected damage is not* the same as actual *damage*. The actual damage is not only affected by what has happened, but also by the internal and external vulnerabilities and resources that the victim of violence has. The actual *damage* we can only know when, for example, we have performed various radiological examinations after a car accident, or have observed our sexually traumatized patient's function, reactions and abilities during assessment and treatment. But risk stratification (a process where patients are divided into risk groups) and assessment help us know what to expect, and what examinations, assessments and treatments we need to have access to in order to be able to offer patient-safe care.

Wonsa has developed a model SAIS (Sexual Abuse Injury Syndrome) that grades sexual traumatization into grades 1–6, where grade six means patients with the highest level of traumatization and one means the lowest level of traumatization. For patients, this is often the first time they encounter therapists, doctors and professionals in a healthcare setting who talk about their abuse as injuries. At level one, there are patients who have been subjected to occasional rape by someone outside the family, and at level six, we find patients who have been subjected to incest throughout their lives, ritual sexual abuse within pedophile circles, trafficking, multiple ACEs, torture or mind control.

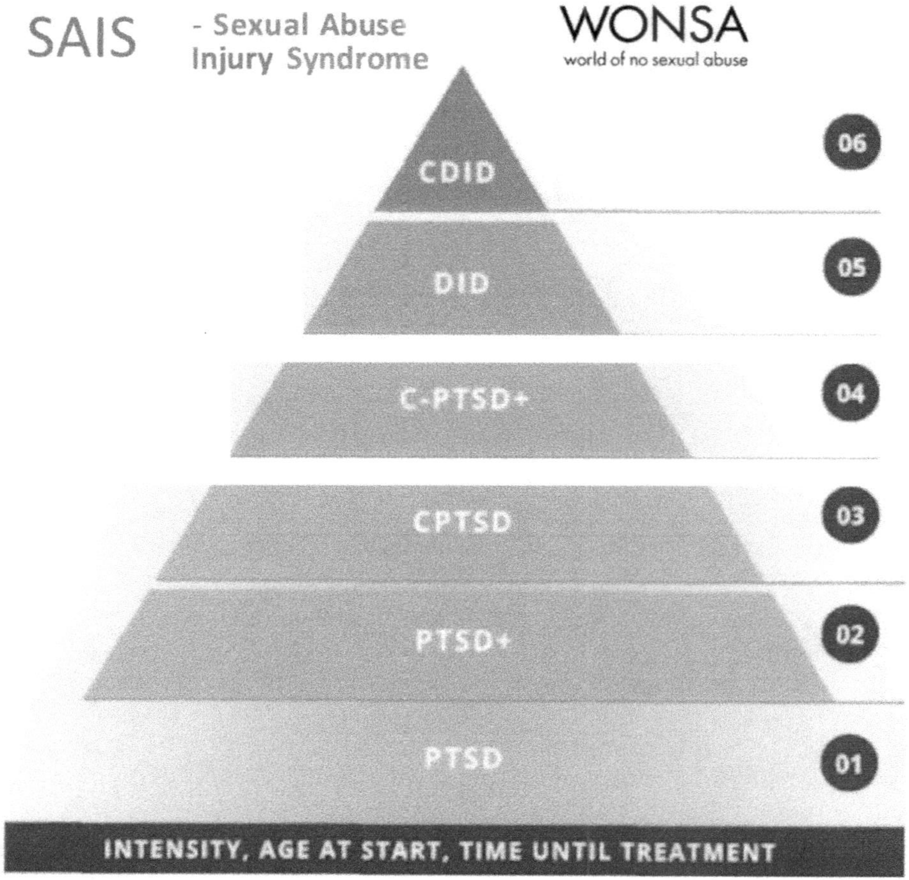

Level 6: Intra-familiare abuse, or large exposure of ACEs, can also be organised abuse, torture or mind-control.
Specialised CDID treatment program.

Level 5: Intra-familiare abuse, or large exposure of ACEs, can also be organised abuse, torture or mind-control.
Specialised DID treatment program.

Level 4: Intra-familiare abuse (incest), or repeated abuse outside family with multiple ACEs. *Four-phase treatment program*

Level 3: Repeated abuse outside family, or few abuses and multiple ACEs.
Four-phase treatment program.

Level 2: one or few type 3 abuses, outside family, with some ACEs.
PTSD-treatment.

Level I: Single type 3. outside family. no or few ACEs. *PTSD-treatment.*

Incest

Incest does not affect a few, it affects many. A meta-analysis examined how childhood sexual abuse is generally reported. The media mainly focuses on perpetrators and detailed descriptions of extreme incidents instead of the common ones. Events are described as isolated, which means that the social aspect and how it affects individuals who are exposed are ignored (Weatherred, 2017). Incest occurs in silence, in the dark, in closed children's rooms where no light reaches. The only witness is the child himself and witness images that can rarely be fully expressed. If the memories ever get words, they are manifested in fragmentary form as loosely connected images without internal chronology, memories of a trauma without a beginning or a clear end.

Rathsman (2001) describes incest as an act of a sexual nature between individuals who are formally or informally related by blood. Incest includes several different variations of abuse such as oral, vaginal, anal sex or penetration with objects in any of these bodily areas by means of threat, force or coercion. Freud (1944) writes in-*Totem and Taboo*, about the incest taboo that he believes has existed throughout time and that regulates who we may and may not experience attraction, desire and sexuality with. He describes how primitive man, with scrupulous accuracy and meticulous rigor, strove to prevent incestuous sexual relations. This prevented members of the same totem from entering into sexual relations or marrying each other. Violation of the prohibition was punished and avenged by the entire tribe as it threatened its survival and entailed a burdensome guilt. Freud argued that the prohibition against incest is the very foundation of our civilization. In this sense, incest becomes not only a crime against a subject, but against all of humanity on a symbolic level. Incest in Sweden has gone from being a religious crime in the 17th century to being considered a violent crime in later centuries. In the 17th–18th centuries, Sweden had the strictest legislation against incest in the world. During the 20th century, there was a change of course after most voluntary incestuous relationships were legalized, and legislators began to take an interest in illicit relationships, especially between fathers and daughters. Clementsson (2017) believes that it was easier to forgive incest between socially equal cousins than between parties who, in theory, should be above and below each other in terms of power. In older times, family ties based on blood ties (kinship) were equated with family ties based on marriage or sexual contacts (brotherhood). Incest was not an ordinary crime of fornication but was counted among the crimes of high morals. These were crimes that were directed against God's own law and such crimes could not be atoned for through secular courts. If one failed to punish such sinners, God could collectively punish the people through accidents, war, crop failure or disease Malmstedt, (1994); referenced in Clementsson, (2017). Incest and sexual abuse have long been a taboo subject in Sweden. People who have been exposed have not dared to talk about the events, citing threats from perpetrators or public opinion. Before the problems were noticed, the blame was placed on the children, as society had a view that girls in particular were seen as loose and seductive. Not telling became a way of protecting oneself (Carlsson, 2009).

Faller (1991) described that during the 1970s, children's accusations of sexual abuse were assumed to be fantasies based on the child's unconscious desires to have a sexual relationship with the adult based on Freud's drive theory. In the early 1990s, there was great interest from clinicians and researchers to further investigate different treatments for dissociation and incest. However, during the same decade, a trend began to grow stronger with a distrust of so-called repressed memories and clinicians who uncovered incest memories, as the number of patients and accusations grew exponentially. There was speculation about suggestion (a psychological influence) and implanted memories by vengeful parents during divorces and by therapists. The memory war was between clinicians who claimed that memories could be repressed and then recovered and researchers who believed that repressed memories did not exist. Clinicians were accused of contaminating patients' memories with false thoughts and ideas. Accusatory, misleading books and articles were written, resulting in a decade of distancing from further research. Between researchers' fear of negative reactions to their work and the general incest taboo, the word incest was almost removed from research contexts. Fonagy (2006) conducted a review of searchable psychoanalytic journals that shows a dramatic decrease in words directly related to sexuality. He cites as a possible explanation a fear of touch among psychodynamicists to distance themselves from the problematic drive theory. The debate remains polarized despite overwhelming research on dissociation. The memory war gained new momentum when therapists began to speak out about organized and ritual abuse revealed by their patients, some leading figures in the issue were sued, and a well-managed media campaign was staged to convince the general population that mind control, ritual, and organized abuse came from the therapist's imagination, not the patient's story (Miller, 2014).

Courtois (2010) distinguishes between incest between blood relatives and incest between an adult and a child who is either legally or by agreement part of the family (marriage to the child's parent, adoption or foster parent) or incest with an adult who is considered close to the family and has a caring function. The degree of abuse of incest is assessed based on the fact that there is a large age difference that generates power and experience. Whether a child has desired, thought about or given consent is irrelevant. Since these are precisely the variables that are created through grooming, coercion or threat by a person with more power. Despite its high prevalence, incestuous behavior is puzzling from an evolutionary perspective. Effects such as inbreeding, depression, increased risk of genetic homozygosity that increases mortality in the offspring of close genetic relatives reduce reproductive fitness, and incest occurs all over the world Charlesworth & Willies, (2009); Seemanová, (1971); referenced in Pullman, Babhishin & Seto, (2019). According to Svedin and Banck (2002), children with disabilities, immigrant children, children from large families, children with previous experience of sexual abuse, and children with many family members are at greater risk of being sexually abused. Children who are sexually abused are often described as lonely, socially isolated, and with few or inadequate peer relationships.

The ruthless, brutal and infinitely harmful nature of abusing children within the family grips you as a therapist. Children who have lost out in the parental lottery suffer on so many different levels in incestuous families. One patient described the effect of many years of exposure to incest as going to war every day. Rapes that occur in adulthood and sexual violence in general also create trauma in the patient, but I have never seen the same damage that incest generates. The complexity of attachment relationships, a body and what should be a safe children's room becomes a crime scene and the knowledge that the same person who abuses the child is the same person who will then comfort, protect and provide care for the child. This very tumble dryer of contradictory emotions creates another dimension of trauma. I usually say that incest spans all fields.

In the book *Our Bodies, Their Battlefields by* Christina Lamb (2020) describes what war does to women in the most horrific conflicts in the world where women and children's bodies have become weapons. Those who are victims of incest recognize the trauma in the story. A hopelessness, total powerlessness of women who have been raped in war, invisible, forgotten, who, unlike the number of dead, cannot be counted. The stigmatization is reminiscent of the shame and guilt that incest survivors describe, but in the children's room battlefield there are no witnesses, only a war that no one saw. Like Lamb's description of brave women who come forward and tell what they have been subjected to, nothing rarely happens in their society. We recognize the experience, incest is allowed to continue year after year and few political proposals, if any, are debated or highlighted. Rapes in war are trivialized and considered tolerable, and incest in turn is relativized and often described in terms of the number of years that the abuse has been going on, no details and no statements.

When Lamb (2020) describes Naima waiting with ten girls for the men from the Islamic State to draw notes about which girl each would take as a slave, Naima comforted the younger, terrified girl next to her by hugging her hand. Several of the incest survivors I met have numerous stories of how they tried to protect their siblings from the abuse. Remaining in the *war even* though they were old enough to move to protect their younger sister or brother. In war, abuse against women and children is systematic with the aim of creating high traumatization. It is said that chaos lives next door to God and that what happens openly in war, happens quietly, in peacetime.

Like the women in Bosnia who were subjected to mass rapes in Sarajevo, those who have survived incest rarely go to the gynecologist and thus have an increased risk of developing cervical cancer. In the 11 conflicts that Lamb respectfully recounts via a witness and rape victim, a survivor from each conflict, the women were often held in camps and the abuse was carried out by one or more perpetrators over a long period of time. Like incest survivors where the average duration of the abuse is 5 years and the median is around 100 rapes. Today in Sweden we have 1-2 children in each classroom who are subjected to systematic rape by perpetrators who in many ways keep the child captive, but we protect ourselves by not talking about it like the war-torn countries that stubbornly refuse to admit that women and children have become weapons in their wars.

Most politicians have a low perception and knowledge of child sexual exploitation and the phenomenon is generally ignored (Briggs, 2012). Schultz (2014) argues that due to the shock and terror that comes with trials dealing with sexual abuse, institutions, government officials and even ministries tasked with protecting children have been whitewashed and their complaints silenced. The worse the abuse, the more entrenched the culture of silence. Organized and ritual sexual abuse of children often has an incest basis (Schröder, Nick, Richter-Appelt & Briken, 2018).

According to the feminist school, the lack of political commitment to address violence against girls stems from cultural contexts and patriarchal structures that imply norms of masculinity and women's submission MacKinnon, (2005); UNICEF, (2000). Today, there is no globally accepted definition of incest, but the meaning of the word is influenced by culture, laws and what is considered acceptable in society. The degree of kinship in relation to the incest taboo also varies, such as marriage between cousins. According to Svedin and Banck (2002), the debate about sexual abuse of children occurs in waves and often intensifies in the media after a case of child pornography, abuse of children in preschool or gang rape has been brought to light. Incest and silence go hand in hand, it often takes decades before a victim get the courage to speak out. But the problem is not the silence of incest survivors, but that we as a society have not listened. Incest as a phenomenon will probably not end, but will always need to be talkable, relevant, and on political agendas. But it's almost as if society is rediscovering this sensitive topic and crime over and over again instead of letting the conversation about incest cease to be taboo once and for all.

A confused dynamic

There are no obvious connections or dividing lines that clearly show whether a family has incestuous relationships. It cuts across race, class, ethnicity, geography and educational levels. Patients with experience of sexual abuse as children are found in all walks of life. However, when examining family dynamics more closely where incest has occurred and generational incest, there are similarities that can increase understanding. In DeYoung & Lowry's study from (1992), the authors demonstrate different explanations and a model for the confusing dynamics involved where incest occurs, as well as in the relationship between the child and the parent. They mention two factors that affect the relationship and interaction between them; the first is the importance of the power relationship between the parent and child and the second is that incest is often periodic with periods of abuse followed by periods where there is no abuse, or loving periods between the parent and the child. To gain a better understanding of the confusing dynamics, the authors suggest that one can look at similar situations that involve a power imbalance and abuse, such as violence in close relationships. In the case of incest, one also needs to take into account the child's dependence on adults, especially their parents. The child's inclination and desire to make an unhappy parent happy constitutes a very unfortunate circumstance for the child in the case of incest (Kvarnmark & Tidefors, 1999). When a parent sexually abuses their child, two essential factors need to be met. The parent is capable of experiencing sexual arousal for their own child and the parent is both psychologically, emotionally and cognitively capable of acting on the experienced sexual arousal. Finkelhor & Araji (1986) explain through a model the confused dynamics that arise before, during and after the abuse.

Phase A is described as a build-up phase, where the parent experiences increased pressure from sexual arousal towards their child. Often the parent tries to reduce the pressure by having sex with, for example, a partner but does not find it sufficiently satisfying. Frustration grows and an initial sexual approach towards the child begins. The parent often rationalizes their behavior and feelings to reduce the cognitive dissonance. The parent initially experiences their feelings as hidden or secret from themselves, and then culminates in openly rationalizing a sexual relationship with their child who is in phase B. A parent in Finkelhor and Araji's study said the following:

When she was about 10, she started to look good to me in a sexual way. I started fantasizing about having sex with her. I started planning it. You see, my wife doesn't really like having sex. She says it feels uncomfortable, like there's something wrong physically, but I know it's mental. So I finally had sex with my daughter, I convinced myself that I was just doing it so she wouldn't have the same problems as her mother. I thought that if I just showed her what sex was about, she wouldn't have the same problems as her mother.

Phase C occurs when the abuse/rape is over and the parent feels a relief from the sexual tension both physically and emotionally. Here, the parent has overcome their original aversion, distaste that created tension, anxiety and frustration. The model shows how the abuse becomes known to both the perpetrator and the victim. The abuse follows a certain procedure. It can be compared to a learning theory for its effectiveness in creating expectations and a behavior that is difficult to remove or end. For the incest victim, it is also divided into the build-up phase, the abuse itself and usually a relief afterwards when the abuse is over. From having been worried and waiting for the next abuse, a brief feeling of calm afterwards occurs. For the parent, there is an increased dependence on the child to reduce their own sexual tension. A traumatic bond for the child has been created. The traumatic bond is described as an emotional dependency between two unequal individuals, an adult and a child, within a relationship that includes periodic sexual abuse. The nature of the relationship includes several dimensions such as feelings of intense attachment, cognitive distortions and behavioral strategies from both parties that paradoxically strengthen and maintain the bond between them. For example, the child actively tries to protect his perpetrator through silence when he understands that the crime is illegal. A secret known only by two creates a symbiosis.

Phase D occurs when the parent may experience shame or guilt for short or long periods when they can no longer rationalize or defend their behavior Roundy and Horton, (1990); referenced in DeYoung and Lowry, (1992). Here, the parent may take on a more appropriate parental role for the child or withdraw from the child. However, as time passes and the parent again experiences increased sexual arousal or tension towards the child, the parent will use the same behavioral strategies to resume the abuse. The abuse becomes a cycle whose repetitive behavior recreates the traumatic bond between the child and the parent (DeYoung & Lowry, 1992). Since the child is not responsible for the abuse or can interpret what motivates it, the child often experiences the abuse as occurring without warning and perceives it as disgusting, punitive, or confusing. A child who is abused will also try to attribute meaning to the abuse, why she is the victim, and to take on blame. But her conclusions will only be as sophisticated as her cognitive development allows (Silver et al., 1983). The young child cannot help but believe that it is my fault that the abuser is doing this to me.

Journal entry woman SAIS grade 4
We do a short exercise and go in and visit the child self (5 years old) and the rabbit Elsa who lives in the nice room we have created together in the imagination. The patient's child self is sitting on the floor and painting. The patient's adult self feels angry that the child self is happy, she does not want to put her arm around her, she describes that she hates herself as a child, she is disgusting and seductive. The patient describes it as karma, she must have been evil in her previous life. We treat a trauma memory where the 5-year-old has been subjected to rape by her father, left alone, confused and terrified. At the end of the exercise, the patient can feel neutral feelings towards herself as a 5-year-old. She manages to tell her younger self that it was not her fault that she played such strange games with her dolls, that was the only thing she knew. But since this does not happen to all children, there must be something wrong with her.

Journal entry woman SAIS 4
The father says during the abuse that *You are more beautiful than your mother, and* I have told her everything and she said nothing. The child feels that the mother sanctions the abuse.

In Nyberg & Dareflod's study from (2010), the build-up phase is described as a worry and anxiety about the expectation that an assault will occur. At nightfall and bedtime, visiting the toilet, bathing and showering, when they knew that they would have to be alone with the perpetrator. The very knowledge that tonight it will happen is something that many of my patients return to, waiting until bedtime, not daring to fall asleep, tensing up, preparing themselves, because afterwards they were left alone, abandoned with the pain, blood, bruises and urinary tract infections as a result of the assault. According to Faller, (1991); Svedin & Banck, (2002), a conflict-filled divorce is considered to entail an increased risk of sexual assault, or false accusations of sexual assault. Faller (1991) states that divorce involves a lack of routines for meals, bedtime, and where the child will sleep, as the structure of the marriage is dissolved. For those who do not want to separate, emotional chaos occurs in the loss of a partner. Anger over the separation can lead parents to regress emotionally and turn to the child as both an object for satisfaction of needs and as retaliation. But it may also be the case that divorce makes it easier for the child to disclose the sexual abuse.

Many victims of extreme sexual abuse refrain from having children and starting a family, consciously or unconsciously, as they associate children with their own abuse and a lifetime of suffering. They may feel a fear that all children will be subjected to horrific abuse. They may also be afraid of being the one to harm the child themselves. A primary agenda for most extreme sexual abuse networks is to force victims to provide them with a new generation of victims. Ritual networks often have long-term agendas of immortality that are based on future generations being able to continue their abuse practices (Lacter, 2022).

Connection

The child develops an attachment system towards the caregivers and the caregivers develop a caregiving system towards the child. Children therefore attach to their parents but parents do not attach to their children. Both systems are genetically pre-programmed. The child is so defenseless when it is born that it would not survive many hours without contact with a caregiver. The child signals its needs for closeness, comfort and protection and the parent responds to the child's signals through one or more caregiving behaviors such as speaking soothingly to the child, picking up the child or hugging the child.

The attachment-care relationship is by definition an unequal relationship, the child receives and the parent gives. The fear system has evolved to protect us and survive in dangerous situations. The fear system includes reactions and behaviors that we call fight/flight, but also freezing of all movement. A child whose one caregiver has been reliably available and whose other caregiver has mostly rejected the child in attachment-relevant situations is likely to develop two very different types of relationships with these caregivers. How a child's attachment to their caregiver develops is largely determined by the type of care the child is offered (Broberg, Granqvist, Ivarsson & Mothander, (2015).

Attachment patterns can be sorted according to two principles; *safe* against *insecure* connection and *organized* against *disorganized attachment*. According to Bowlby (1973), an important signal of insecure attachment is that the child shows aggression. Insecure avoidant attachment is more about how the child greets the parent upon reunion rather than whether they cry when the parent leaves the room. Here, the child does not use the parent as a secure base but avoids contact with the parent when the parent enters the room after a separation. The child can often handle separations without crying, may look down and avoid eye contact with the parent or turn their back on the parent. Insecure ambivalent/resisting attachment instead shows a maximized need for attachment and the child becomes very upset when the parent leaves the room. Some lie completely exhausted on the floor while others stand kicking and screaming at the door. The decisive factor for classification is how the child acts upon reunion with parents. The problem with insecure ambivalent attachment is that contact with the parent is not effective, which means that the relationship does not allow the child's attachment system to rest. By being anxious, monitoring every step the parent takes, and by clinging to the parent, the child acquires the closeness it needs to be guaranteed protection if real danger threatens. I remember a parent in therapy who found it amusing to hide outside in public settings at shopping malls and bus stops for her 5-year-old child until the child was beside himself with despair and fear, and then emerge and tell him that it was not so dangerous. Her son never left her side.

In disoriented attachment, Main & Solomon, (1986); (1990); referenced in Broberg, Granqvist, Ivarsson & Risholm Mothander, (2015) believe that the relationship between the child and the parent is largely based on fear. Bowlby described it in the early 1950s as a chronically switched-on attachment system. This means that the child's attachment system is activated at the same time as there is no secure adult who can help the child regain security so that the attachment system can be put into hibernation. In disoriented attachment, the child may exhibit strange behaviors such as hiding behind a chair, walking with their back to the parent, putting their hands in front of their face when the parent enters the room (as if to protect themselves), freezing their behavior in the middle of a movement and becoming completely still for a moment when the parent approaches, and displaying various types of behaviors such as waving their hands in the air or banging their head against the wall. When the person who is supposed to be a protective adult is the same person who activates the child's attachment system by arousing fear in the child and acting threateningly, an impossible conflict situation is created for the child Broberg, Granqvist, Ivarsson & Risholm Mothander; (2015). According to Main & Solomon (1990); referenced in Greenfield (2012), threatening and frightening childhood experiences carried out by an attachment figure on whom the child is dependent are too overwhelming to be integrated and thus need to remain segregated. A fear without a solution.

The vast majority of traumatized patients have disoriented, unresolved attachment patterns with unresolved conflicts between closeness and distance. One part of the patient moves towards wanting to approach while the other part engages in fight/flight or immobilization defenses such as freeze and collapse. Disorganized attachment patterns have been shown to be associated with chronic dissociation and dissociative diagnoses during development (Boon, 2016).

Possible motives for incest

Maddock & Larson (1995) set out to explain the motives that may lie behind families where incest occurs. They divided different incestuous family dynamics into; a) *Affect-based*, incest creates a closeness in the family that otherwise lacks a caring and emotional approach towards each other. Here the focus is on a feeling of being special in the relationship that otherwise fails through unavailability and inability to be caring; b) *Erotica-based incest* means that the family atmosphere resembles a chaotic pansexual one and it is not uncommon for several members to be involved in the incest. An eroticization of relationships similar to polyincest with many perpetrators; c) *Aggression-based incest*, here the incest consists of the perpetrator's sexualized contempt and anger. The perpetrator vents his frustration and conflicts on a vulnerable individual, psychological abuse often occurs; d) *Furious incest* means that the perpetrator is threatening and has sadistic traits. For the victim, it means a great danger to his life. According to Kluft (2010), it is not uncommon for the different motives to be mixed and changed over time. He also addresses incestuous relationships without physical abuse where a parent intrudes and uses the child as a surrogate partner, who becomes trapped in a world dominated by a parent. These relationships are often seductive in nature and are called *emotional incest*. There are also hypotheses that highlight that family structures are different in families where incest occurs. Seto et al., (2015) mention that clinicians and other therapists have reported on beliefs, attitudes and dynamics in the family as possible explanatory models. They refer to a belief in family structures where incest occurs, that there is a belief that incest does not harm the child or that the child can even benefit from being abused by an adult. The study shows that the generational trauma where incest is passed from one generation to another has often had a deficient attachment to the child and deficient relationships between mother and daughter, families where the parents have problems in marriage, low levels of satisfaction, violence in close relationships with the mother as the victim, higher tolerance of nudity between the father and daughter, being separated from their siblings for more than two years before the age of six, low income, single parent with a new partner and various types of abuse. Since incest is often found in family structures with multiple traumatic childhood experiences, ACS:s and neglect, the child has often not learned to take care of his basic physical care. In some families, the child does not learn to take care of his body, for example to prevent diseases, to eat healthy and exercise, to have regular check-ups with the dentist or doctor. Without these abilities, they need to be learned in adulthood through practice, attention and training. But we need to keep in mind that those exposed to incest are not a homogeneous group, explanatory models always need to take into account the complex dynamics that incest entails.

Seto (2015) divides the factors that motivate perpetrators to commit child abuse into two dimensions. If an individual has deviant sexual behavior such as a paraphilia, this can be a motivating factor to seek out children for sexual purposes. As well as if a person has antisocial tendencies that include impulsivity, insensitivity or increased risk-taking. This theory has been supported by several studies and meta-analyses conducted on childhood sexual abuse (Hawes et al., 2013). However, what is a mystery is that perpetrators within the family, as in the case of incest, do not exhibit antisocial tendencies or atypical sexual tendencies to a greater extent than men who are not perpetrators (Chaplin, et al., 1995). This means that it is difficult to detect incest based on the fact that perpetrators do not exhibit antisocial behavior. We cannot look at someone to see if they are a perpetrator, in many cases the only witness is the child. This should also take the blame away from mothers who did not discover the incest. But despite the fact that the perpetrator is almost always a man and many mothers testify to having been completely unaware, Jensen, (2005); referenced in Pettersen, (2013) argues that maternal blame is so strong that it exists among survivors despite the fact that many mothers support their children after the sexual abuse is revealed.

Resistance always exists

If we put our ear to the ground and examine the details of an assault, we will come to the realization that resistance has occurred. Burstow & Weitz, (1988); Coates et al., (2003); Haig-Brown, (1988) argue that victims always resist violence and other forms of abuse. Thus, alongside every story of violence, there is a story of well-considered, resolute and often creative resistance (Wade, 1997). How the victim resists depends on the unique combination of risks and opportunities in each given situation. The victim needs to take into account that the perpetrator may become even more violent if they are met with defiance. Open defiance on the part of the victim is therefore the least common form of resistance (Burstow & Weitz, 1988). In extreme cases, the only possibility for the victim to resist may be to do so in their minds. The victim can resist in a variety of ways that can lead to the violence ending or being prevented, but this is often not the case. In the therapy room, I always raise the question of how they resisted, as the knowledge of the power of resistance is healing with expressions of dignity and self-respect. At first, the question may seem difficult to understand. They imagine that the resistance must have been loud, violent or powerful. When we investigate, we find small signs of conscious resistance. As children, they have withdrawn, walked outside for hours, run away to the stable, got boyfriends to sleep away, refused gifts and bribes, pressed their legs together, been passive during the abuse, not showered for days, stopped calling their parent dad, slept with their clothes on, kept things a secret, wrapped the covers tightly around their bodies at bedtime and told their friends about their hatred and contempt for the perpetrators. Small, small deeds that when we talk about them give the patient back even a ounce of self-respect. He took my body but he could never take over my thoughts. As psychotherapists, we have an important role to recognize and pay attention to the spontaneous resistance that the child has demonstrated to show the patient that they have not been passive but have actively tried to change their situation. The very knowledge that you have actually resisted means that you also understand that it was not my fault. When you show the resistance, it means that I was not involved in it. You have not participated if you have resisted, it becomes the antithesis of willing participation.

Journal entry woman SAIS 6 DID
The patient has sent a drawing with various speech bubbles to the part I know is that I fought it, I didn't want this. If I make it, I'm going to make sure no child has to go through this. I'm going to get through this, it's not worth letting him destroy me. Every damn piece is going back where it belongs.

Incest in culture

According to Seidel (1991), the perpetrator parent may favor the child who is being abused. This can lead to the parent acting with jealousy and becoming controlling when the child is in contact with others, such as a potential girlfriend or boyfriend. Sometimes other family members may feel jealous of the favored child. According to Seidel, strong jealous reactions can be an indicator that abuse is occurring in the family. In the HBO documentary about the allegations against Woody Allen, Dylan Farrow talks about the sexual abuse she accuses him of having subjected her to when she was 7 years old. She describes that Allan showed strong jealousy, overly protectiveness and inappropriate physical closeness in both abusive situations but mainly in everyday situations. The documentary shows private videos that have never before been shown of how Allen follows Farrow everywhere, always has her on his lap and touches her like a jealous stalking partner. Culture sometimes tries to portray the confused dynamics and victims who don't always behave as we think or expect. In the Israeli film*That lovely girl* by Keren Yedayas depicts the incestuous destructive relationship between the father who is 50 years old and the daughter who is 20 years old. She mostly stays indoors and struggles with his bulimia and self-hatred. Until the day the father brings home a girlfriend her own age and the daughter goes crazy with jealousy and envy and storms out and seeks out new situations in which she is exploited. Also in the film, Dalva by Emmanuelle Nicot describes a 12-year-old girl who feels completely misunderstood and abandoned when she is picked up in the middle of the night by the police and social services and separated from the love of her life, her father, Jacques. Her father has just been taken into care by the authorities for abusing her. In the beginning of the film, she walks around her new home in small pumps, cocktail dresses, dressed up and lipstick, she tries to escape to be reunited with him. The confused dynamics that exist in incestuous families can seem incomprehensible to outsiders who are not woven into the deceitful family secrets. In Thomas Vinterberg's dogmatic film Festen från (1998), we follow Christian who has traveled home from Paris to attend his father's 60th birthday party. The guests have been invited to the family estate and at dinner Christian clinks his glasses and begins to tell an everyday story about how he and his late twin sister played as children. Then he goes on to describe how his father always wanted to bathe together. Or that the twins would play in his office, he locked the door, took off his clothes and raped us on the couch, sexually exploited us. He was a very clean man. Christian then describes his mother's denial by giving a speech. Uh...in 1974, you, my mother, came into the office and saw your son standing on all fours and your husband was without pants. I'm sorry that you had to see your son like that, that your husband asked you to leave and that you did. I'm sorry that you are so deceitful and rotten. When the shaky camera zooms in on the mother's face, who has actively tried to convince the guests throughout the evening that Christian is sick and has a vivid imagination, breathing stops for a short moment. You can feel the atmosphere as the family's dirty secrets come to light. Thank you for all the good years, Christian concludes his speech. Someone starts clapping their hands in confusion, the father drinks a toast and, together with the guests, manages to cover up what has actually been said. In Vinterberg's chamber play, it is not the fine people in the bright rooms who are left to stand for civil courage and truth, but the servants in the dark spaces, those who have witnessed the abuses (Granath, 1998).

Culture portrays incest based on the legislation and culture of its society. In recent years, France has been shaken by a series of pedophile and incest scandals that extend all the way to the top of society. France has been criticized for not having a clear lower age for sexual intercourse that is considered rape. A person under 15 is considered a minor, but age has not been considered the only criterion for it to be considered rape. As recently as (1977), several of the most prominent French intellectuals of the time: Simone de Beauvoir, Jean-Paul Sartre, Roland Barthes, Gilles Deleuze, Louis Aragon,

Louis Althusser, Michael Foucault, Jacques Derrida and child psychologist Francoise Dolto wrote an open letter demanding that the law against sexual relations between adults and minors be abolished (referenced in GP). Philosopher Micael Foucault is one of France's greatest thinkers, he was accused (2021) by Guy Sorman of raping children in Tunisia in the 1960s. Foucault has been dead for several decades and cannot defend himself, but the accusations against him have shaken the upper echelons of society and several philosophers and colleagues have come to his defense. Foucault is an icon for French left-wing intellectuals, for his groundbreaking analyses of power, madness and sexuality. Guy Sorman, who accused Foucault when he was interviewed on the program C ce Soir on French TV, has been honored with the Legion of Honor, France's highest order, in a country where philosophers are celebrated like rock stars. Sorman claims that it is now time to reveal the truth of the greatest of them all, that Foucault was the royal philosopher. He believes that France has now entered a new era where there is no longer a moral yardstick for the aristocracy and one for the people. Gabriel Matzneff is another French author who, in his books, romanticized and glorified sexual relations with children for decades, until (2023) he was reported to the police for pedophilia after one of his victims came forward (referenced in SvD).

Child sexual abuse material

Ireland has replaced the general term *child pornography* with *child sexual abuse material.* They argue that the term child pornography is outdated, inappropriate and fails to reflect the real torture and horror that sexual abuse of a child generates. A sexual image of a child is an abuse and not pornography and should therefore be described as an abuse. Pornography is a term for adults who engage in sex with consent (mostly) legally for the general public for sexual pleasure. Images of children being raped therefore do not fall into the same category (The Journal, 2025). We live in a world where abuse is no longer something that happens behind closed doors, in children's rooms or in closed societies. Today, pedophiles and pedophile networks choose to openly document, disseminate, share and create digital material that circulates, every second, minute, hour, day, month and year. The evidence of violent abuse of children is endless. The image and film material that is reviewed by the Police is of varying nature. Everything from simple nude and posing pictures to films, depictions of sexual acts and gross sexual abuse, torture and violence. According to Ahlénius, (2006); Nilsson, (2003); referenced in Jameson, (2007), individual seizures of over 100,000 pictures are not uncommon in this context. Netclean (2015) investigated child pornography crimes by asking 368 police officers who work with the issue on a daily basis from 28 countries about their experiences. Of these, 97% responded that their working situation had become more demanding in the past year. The reason given by 80% was that they handle more and more cases and more material per case. The survey shows that 81% of the police officers say that the amount of pictures and films showing sexual abuse of children has increased in the past three years, 43% of the police officers testify that the abuse has become more serious. The police are continuously receiving large amounts of images and films captured by social media services that may constitute abuse material. The material that comes in via an American organization is screened centrally to find the most serious and urgent cases, such as people who have filmed their own abuse or where the sender has their own children or works with children. Then there is a large amount that needs to be checked more thoroughly to see if it is about possession or dissemination of abuse. In the article*The price for raping a child: 150 SEK* in DN, (2025) describes the Philippines as the world's epicenter for child sexual abuse, as almost everyone uses the internet and speaks English. Every year, an estimated half a million Filipino children are exploited for sexual purposes. The Swedish police interviewed in the article describe that there are no barriers in this world and that the children are completely numb. In the article, the police describe that the children who are exposed have rarely experienced any other reality and that both the client and the perpetrator want the business to continue. The children are often sold to several different countries at the same time, as they have already developed a dissociative basis. The American investigative unit Homeland Security Investigations (HSI) plays a key role in the international fight against the rape industry. Sweden is a small country but is one of those that stands out regarding money transactions and suspected perpetrators, according to American intelligence information. They describe to DN that the Swedish perpetrators stand out when they have ordered "*some of the most heinous abuses*".

According to Miller (2014), we can speculate that pedophile groups that create child pornography often borrow children from multi-generational incestuous families, as these children already have a dissociative basis. Organized pedophile circles know that the child's dissociation is the key to maintaining power and secrets. Miller further claims that almost all of her over 1000 patients she has treated in organized and ritual abuse in the United States report that they were also used in child prostitution and child pornography. Lucas (2022) writes that children in organized sexual abuse are often forced to commit sexual abuse against other children, which is then filmed and used to blackmail the child into committing more abuse by threatening to show the films to the police. Of 165 individuals in Schröder, Nick, Richter-Appelt and Briken's study from (2018) where the participants themselves estimated that they had experienced organized and ritual abuse as children, 66.7% had been in child prostitution, 64.8% had recorded child pornography and/or violent pornography. According to Lacter (2022), networks that produce child rape and torture use girls who are too old to accommodate new younger girls for the network. They often force the children to harm and abuse other children who they then film and threaten to hand them over to the authorities if the victims do not do as they say and follow directives that then include giving other girls access to child pornography. Goldberg (2025) from the organization Not Standing Idle By describes that the perpetrators deceive the children and are so cruel to them that it is difficult to accept. But that the cruelties at a later stage benefit the perpetrators since no one believes that what the victims say is the truth. Her organization has watched several films in which children are gang-raped by adult men and sometimes women. The films involve drugs, ritual practices and symbolism (The Jerusalem Post).

AI identifies vulnerable children

The police have become better at identifying children who are victims of documented sexual crimes. Through AI, the police have moved from looking at image by image to focusing on finding children who are being victimized in the present. When they identify a child, social services are contacted to be able to provide the children with the right support. But above all, if they find the children, they find the perpetrator and have secured evidence through documented material. The police work with their own analysis program with effective AI functions, partly with an Interpol database to which around 70 countries are connected. This means that images and films of already identified children do not need to be searched for and worked with again. Instead, the police can focus on identifying new, unknown children by analyzing traces in images and films. This can involve looking in the visual for clues around the crime scene. Previously, it was like looking for a needle in a haystack, but with smarter methods, the police can search for children who are exposed to serious crimes more quickly, more efficiently, with less risk of secondary traumatization, and prosecute the perpetrators (Polisen 2025). There are hopes that adult victims, together with the Police, will in the future be able to search for images and film material circulating about themselves as children in order to secure evidence and obtain legal redress.

Detecting sexual abuse of young children

There are signs that staff should be trained in, which are a collective knowledge of how to detect sexual abuse of young children. Sexual abuse of children causes few if any physical injuries, but mainly injuries that are not visible. Only a few of the children who have been exposed to penetrative sexual abuse have injuries that can be detected during a medical examination of the genitals and anus. This is because children heal quickly and there is often a long time between the abuse and the examination. But it is also because the abuse usually does not lead to visible physical injuries (Kastbom, 2016).

Physical signs of child sexual abuse

Recurrent discomfort or pain in the throat and pharynx, redness, bleeding or bruising of the palate or tears in the corners of the mouth or pharynx. May occur with repeated oral abuse.
Redness, swelling and bleeding in the genital area, damage to the internal parts of the genitals or damage to the anal area, such as redness and cracks.
Grip marks on thighs or buttocks. Several oval bruises in a row can be a sign of a hard grip. Sometimes grip marks are seen on the inner thighs or buttocks. This is a place where children rarely hit themselves and get bruises.
Crescent-shaped wounds behind the ears. Caused by fingernails after a tight grip on the child's head when the child is forced to perform oral sex.

Recurrent urinary tract infections.
Infections in the genitals caused by sexually transmitted infections. This is very uncommon but strongly indicates that abuse has occurred. Symptoms to look out for include pain in the genitals, especially when the child urinates, and if the child has vaginal discharge Dahlström – Lannes, (1994); National Handbook of Child Health Care, (2017).

Mangilio, (2009); Righthand et al., (2003); Sanderson, (2004); referenced in the Child Safety Practice Manual (2025) address the following indicators of child sexual abuse:

Physiological indicators

Bruising, bleeding, swelling, scrapes, or cuts on the genitals or anus
An unusual vaginal odor or discharge
Teary, stained, blood on clothes, difficulty going to the bathroom, walking or sitting
Sexually transmitted diseases or infections, especially before adolescence and pregnancy

Emotional indicators, sudden changes within:

Anxiety
Arousal (excitement/activation) anxious, unusually fearful or cautious
Changes in mood
Depression
Feelings of hopelessness or feelings of helplessness
Fear of specific situations, people, or things
Insensibility
Hyperactivity
Intense fear
Difficulty concentrating
Lethargy and apathy
Memory problems
Nightmares, difficulty sleeping and fear of the dark

Behavioral indicators- Sexual

Self-harm behavior
Has or is involved with many sexual partners
Early sexual debut and sexual behavior
Sexual behavior that is unexpected or developmentally inappropriate
Hiding intimate items such as underwear, bras, used tampons or pads
Suicide attempts or accidents involving fire in places where abuse is alleged to have occurred
Placing objects in the genitals
Smears feces or blood on their body

General behavioral indicators

Aggressiveness	Avoidance of people or places
Bedwetting	Privacy
Drug or alcohol use	Vaghet
Eating disorders, difficulty swallowing	Losing control over eating
Oppositional or defiant	Physical pain
Flashbacks or nightmares	School refusal, truancy or school-related problems

Self-harm behavior	Sleep problems
Insulation	Social problems
Pulling away	Conflicts with peers
Theft	Suicidal thoughts
Running away from home	Gets an outbreak
Potty training problems	

As a therapist for patients with early sexual abuse, we usually order the patient's medical records from the regional archive and social services together. The patients have often received treatment for their injuries caused by the sexual abuse, but almost never is there any mention of suspicion of sexual abuse in the medical records. Here are some examples from adult patients with experience of incest and ritual sexual abuse as children.

Journal entry woman SAIS 4
The medical records from the region show multiple hospitalizations (5-7 years) and urinary tract infections that at one point progressed to the kidneys and led to surgery.

Journal entry woman SAIS 5
The patient tested positive for chlamydia as a child.

Journal entry woman SAIS 4
The medical records show that the patient's internal organs continue to move as an infant, as well as ulcers in her lower abdomen. The doctor prescribes ointment.

Journal entry woman SAIS 5
The medical record shows that the doctor experiences the patient's abdomen as red.

Journal entry woman SAIS 6 DID
The patient shows photographs of herself as a child when she was about 2-8 years old. She has bruises around her mouth and sores at the corners of her mouth.

Journal entry woman SAIS 6 DID
The patient regains memories of ritual abuse that she was cut in the lower abdomen. She visits a gynecologist as an adult. Excerpt from the medical record: Vulva with thin scars, one on the right side and one on the left side, lateral to the labia 3 cm scar on the left side and 4 cm on the right side.

Journal entry woman SAIS 6 DID
Pat has several memories of having broken ribs when she was revived during ritual abuse involving strangulation, heavy medication and being forced under water by her perpetrators. As an adult, she visits her VC and asks for an examination and X-ray. The medical record shows the following: Pat reports pain in the lower ribs on the right side and right shoulder. Pat has a swelling on the right side of about 7-8 cm which probably comes from a previous fracture. Pat reports 16 resuscitation attempts. The clinical examination shows; right shoulder swelling of 3-5 cm on the acromioclavicular joint (a small joint between the collarbone and the shoulder blade).

Journal entry woman SAIS 4
Pat is a teenager and lives with an older man who subjected her to severe rapes for about 2 years. She seeks medical help on several occasions for cracks in her vagina, she develops vaginismus. The man often accompanies her to the gynecologit and doctor visits, which makes her afraid and prevents her from talking about the violence and rapes.

Journal entry woman SAIS 5 DID
The patient sends photographs of over 60 scars all over his body that were caused during ritual sexual abuse.

According to Svedin & Banck (2002), it is important to be aware of the child's normal development because sexualized behavior is a natural part of children's development.

This makes it easier to identify which type of behavior occurs within the framework of normal development and which does not. The sexual maturation process includes curiosity, sexually charged games and experiments where the child can test role models that occur in the surrounding society. According to Tidefors, Andersson, (2002), it is obvious that children have the right to be sexual and seductive in different phases of their development. The child's sexual curiosity and sexual exploration have nothing to do with incest. Incest occurs when sexual reactions are aroused in the parent and these are acted out towards the child. In the same way, children can behave seductively towards other adults, which must not be exploited by the adult. According to Save the Children (2016), sexual abuse during childhood can lead to sexualized problem behavior where the victim exposes other children to sexual transgressions. Children's sexual behavior becomes problematic when the play is characterized by coercion, threats or violence. The behavior is compulsive, driven by anxiety and difficult for the adult to interrupt. Many of my patients testify to compulsive sexualized behavior as children, through self-stimulation of the genitals, rubbing themselves against objects or forcing themselves on peers and siblings. It is complex how the child shows signals and signs of abuse, sometimes it can involve behavioral disorders such as regression, that the child goes backward in their development (Lingåker, 2017).

The Disclosure - Receiving a Story

When a child chooses to talk about sexual abuse to an educator, it is the educator's task to let the child tell the story, show interest in the child's story and show that they believe the child (Swedish National Board of Health and Welfare, 2010). A basic rule is to let the child tell the story but not to ask more than necessary (Dahlström-Lannes 1994). Gustavsson (2011) points out that the adult needs to be aware of their approach in conversations when the child is telling the story and use language that the child understands, explain terms, listen, have a neutral approach and be flexible in their thinking about the child's situation and experience. As a preschool educator, you need to listen and pay attention to the signals and signs of vulnerable children. The social discourse surrounding incest and sexual abuse means that the story is frequently questioned both in terms of credibility and that survivors are accused of having poor judgment and inappropriate behavior. This in turn leads to internalization that negatively affects the rehabilitation process, avoiding seeking help, social isolation and negative self-image with guilt and shame as a result Kennedy et al., (2012); Kennedy & Prock, (2018); referenced in Shaked, Benisimon & Mashiack, (2021). Patients exposed to sexual violence in childhood need a therapist whose reality includes a conceptual world that there is such pure and simple indifference that perpetrators show. One patient said that it is so nice that you can understand that there are such sick people like my father. Since incest is associated with shame, guilt and protecting secrets, it is a complicated process for the victim to talk about their experiences. Traumatic memories consist of images, sensations, emotional states and behaviors that are constant and remain unchanged over time. They can arouse panic, rage, shame, loss, guilt, despair, contradictory beliefs or thoughts (Boon, Steele, Van Der Hart, 2012). The memories are state-dependent and cannot be evoked by the patient's will, not arranged in such a way that they cope with social expectations, which means that the listener needs to be patient when receiving the story. The story will be fragmented, sometimes not perceived as consistent and does not follow a given time order. According to Svedin & Banck (2002), the child's storytelling will appear as a process, where the child reads the adult's reactions and investigates whether there is trust. The child may begin by suggesting that there is a secret. According to Dahlström-Lannes (1994), it is natural to be upset when learning about sexual abuse, but it is important to maintain a neutral approach, especially since young children do not yet know what is right or wrong. The child may take back their story if the person they confided in acts skeptically or becomes upset. Telling someone else can both hinder and facilitate healing. It depends on how they are treated.

According to Bird (2018), it is valuable for children to learn rules around the concept of sexual consent from a young age. She believes that if children receive information in a pedagogically adapted way, a discussion on the subject can start as early as three years of age. But then with explanations that they understand. When it comes to sexual abuse, this does not occur to any great extent, Bird believes, which is problematic. According to Svensson (2007), children's books have a great influence on children and convey factual knowledge, social skills, ethical values and personal development. In the children's book *The Octopus by* Dahle & Nyhus (2017) the authors tell about little Gullet who has a door that she can close when she wants to be alone, until the octopus comes and locks them both in. He breathes so strangely and little Gullet stops shining and sparkling because she is no longer a nugget of gold. The authors describe the art of writing to a child without paraphrasing or lying about secrets that you are not allowed to speak or tell. The story shows that if the child tells about the octopus it stops being dangerous and little Gullet will start sparkling again. You don't have to carry your secret your whole life.

Sgori et al., (1982) describe how the process intensifies when a perpetrator approaches a child. In step a) *engagement*, the relationship between the perpetrator and the victim intensifies. The child is involved in gradually more sexualized behavior through attention and the perpetrator's involvement in the child's emotional needs. Sexualization is often introduced through play and activities that the child initially shows interest in. Some perpetrators use violence or threats to force sexual involvement. In stage b) *the sexual interaction phase*, The perpetrator builds on the initial grooming of the victim and initiates several sexual acts that escalate, often going from posing and caressing to various forms of penetration. In step c) *secrecy*, the perpetrator assures the victim that they will remain silent about the abuse, this is done by making the child complicit and responsible for the abuse. The child is made aware that a disclosure will cause very serious consequences. The agreement often includes threats to harm the child or others. The threat consists of a loss of attachment figures, telling the child that no one will believe the child, saying that the child liked what happened. This confusion or brainwashing of the child leads to self-hatred, a belief that she is evil, that disclosure would confirm her incompetence and guaranteed displacement. In step d) *disclosure*, the secret comes to light, either spontaneously, by accident or deliberately. How the disclosure is received in the family depends on the role of the perpetrator in the family structure. The family's honor/loyalty or shame becomes prominent rather than what is best for the child in question. Families tend to be more positive about a disclosure when the perpetrator is not a parent or sibling. In an attempt to protect the family, family members tend to minimize the seriousness of the crime or blame the victim and other professionals involved. A protection of the perpetrator who is *one of us can* lead to the family blaming the victim by attacking the authenticity of the statement. This results in the patient's world being turned upside down when a disclosure occurs in the therapy room, doctor's office, or social services. Conflicts of loyalty for the victim can be more traumatic than the trauma itself. In step e) *suppression*, the environment and individuals in the family structure will try to influence the credibility of the story by minimizing both the seriousness of the abuse and its consequences. The family does not want to accept the disgusting truth and is eager to try to escape the shame and discomfort that the disclosure creates. Individuals can actively try to influence the victim to retract their statement. If you side with the perpetrator, you do not need to do anything, but if you choose the victim, it requires action.

A survivor often has many hours of preparation, thinking and worry before they eventually choose to tell someone about what they have been exposed to. How they choose to disclose has been identified in different categories.

Conscious storytelling, when the person tells with the intention of telling
Unconscious storytelling, when the person tells without being aware of it, happens to tell
Evoked or prompted storytelling, when the person tells after being asked
Behavioral storytelling, when the person tells stories with their behavior, non-verbal communication
Deliberate non-telling, the person deliberately withholds information, a choice not to tell, denial of what happened
Triggered to tell, when the person tells fragments, has flashbacks, repressed memories

Storytelling rarely follows a linear process but may involve several different types of storytelling before the whole story is conveyed. What prevents a child from telling in the present may be shame, embarrassment, dysfunction in the family, fear of what will happen to the perpetrator, a desire to protect certain family members, or a lack of conscious memories. When an adult chooses to tell about experiences of childhood sexual abuse, disclosure is often referred to as giving someone a trust (Berliner & Elliott, 2002).

A doctoral dissertation examined how women disclose experiences of sexual abuse and the importance of the treatment for their recovery and healing. Telling the truth was described as the most difficult and most frightening way. It required that they felt completely ready to tell. Reasons that prevented respondents from telling were previous experiences of people who refused to listen, encouraged them to forget, did not believe them or that they had told people who then committed new abuses on them. The results showed that being denied a disclosure means being denied a part of one's life and identity. Which becomes an extension of the trauma with new secrets that constantly intrude. Disclosure becomes counter-power. When it is not possible to talk about one's experiences, the body tells the story, through the body the experiences of violence leak out and claim their right to be included (Graham, Dickerson, 2001). Anyone who has been sexually exploited, oppressed or harmed by another person has the right to redress and legal justice. This means that every individual should be able to receive redress or compensation in a legal sense, that what has been done wrong to her is brought to light and corrected. But before that can happen, the victim needs to report and the court needs to judge the acts committed against the victim. In the case of sexual abuse, there are rarely any witnesses other than the victim and the perpetrator, and it is almost impossible to obtain redress and justice after sexual abuse. Most vulnerable children do not disclose the abuse at the time and therefore do not receive any help. Swedish and international studies show that victims of crime fall away at different stages. The first stage means that children do not disclose abuse in the immediate aftermath of it, where half of them fall away. Many of the victims tell their stories decades later in treatment or when they participate in a research study. Of the minority who do disclose, 6–12% are reported to the authorities. In only 1% of cases is it as a result of an offender confessing. The study shows that only 5% of police reports lead to prosecution and half of them to conviction (Svedin, 1999). With these figures, it becomes obvious that part of the healing lies in the response, the listening and the disclosure being well received.

Journal entry woman SAIS 4

When the patient tells her guardian what happened, she is told that she can take it to her grandfather herself.

How sexual abuse affects health as an adult

We humans are not our diagnoses and symptoms, but we have assumed them for reasons and meaning. If you try to find a living story, delve into a person's life history, upbringing, illness and the relationships around the person, the context for a deeper understanding emerges Palle Villemoes, (1993); referenced in Svaleklint, (2014). Unlike adults, children, when they are exposed to sexual abuse, are always in a critical period of their development Svedin and Banck, (2002). According to Roberts et al., (2004), victims of incest are at higher risk for several negative consequences in life such as poorer psychological well-being, feeling broken and suffering from depression, being estranged from one or both parents, higher risk of teenage pregnancy, experiencing sexual ill health as adults, lower socioeconomic status as adults than other victims of childhood sexual abuse. Children and young people who are exposed to sexual abuse experience psychological symptoms such as difficulty concentrating, guilt and shame, self-destructiveness, depression, anxiety, worry and fear, psychosis, suicidal thoughts, sleep problems, etc. Children who are exposed to sexual abuse are at greater risk of suffering from pain symptoms such as chronic pelvic pain, muscle pain, headaches and stomach and intestinal problems (Poleshuck et al., 2009). Almost all survivors of incest experience mental stress that negatively affects the individual such as PTSD (post-traumatic stress disorder), depression, eating disorders Gur, (2019); referenced in Shaked, Benismon & Mashiach, (2021), psychotic episodes, including schizophrenia and personality disorders Cujatar et al., (2010); referenced in Shaked, Benismon & Mashiach, (2021). In addition, adult survivors of incest may suffer from chronic effects on multiple psychological systems as well as severe illnesses and conditions, some of which cannot be explained medically Anda et al., (2006); Feletti et al., (1998). Confirmed correlated effects include impaired immune function, gynecological and reproductive problems, difficulty urinating, gastroscopic problems, cardiovascular diseases, cancer, liver diseases, obesity, headaches, generalized musculoskeletal pain Bohn & Holz, (1996); Mulvihill, (2005); Runtz, (2002); Sachs-Ericson et al., (2005); referenced in Shaked, Benismon & Mashiach, (2021). This means that patients with experiences of incest and sexual abuse are found in both psychiatric and somatic care. Many of Wonsa's patients describe sometimes hopeless attempts for decades in their quest to find the right care provider and be understood. Rape causes psychological damage that can be treated, but there is currently a lack of treatment facilities and specialist expertise (WONSA, 2023).

Patients who have been subjected to trafficking, organized and ritual sexual abuse are found across the spectrum of healthcare and welfare systems, and they often have complex trauma-related dissociative symptoms. Their symptoms often exceed the clinical criteria for PTSD, primarily regarding interpersonal disturbances, negative self-image and major problems with affect regulation. Individuals with CPTSD often have higher scores on dissociation scales than those with PTSD. Dissociation is also related to fear of relationships and withdrawal from situations that may arouse feelings of shame (Schröder, Nick, Richter-Appelt, & Briken, 2018).

In one of the first studies to examine the long-term effects of women who have been exposed to incest, Putnam & Trickett (1986) came to general findings that had previously only been reported by individual incest survivors. The study showed how female incest survivors mature in relation to their non-exposed peers in terms of peer relationships, self-concept, and how they later interact with partners. Exposed children have a different developmental curve in several aspects of life than non-exposed children. They often lack friends of the same age due to the feeling that no one can be trusted. Self-loathing and self-hatred is common when the biological changes that occur naturally are against them, many times the child overreacts to simpler stimuli or shuts down completely. Common age-appropriate games that deal with envy, inclusion, exclusion that require staying calm under stress become particularly challenging. Girls who have been exposed to incest mature sexually and reach puberty about 18 months before non-exposed girls. Sexual abuse speeds up the biological clock and releases pubertal hormones. Girls who have been abused have 3–5 times higher levels of testosterone, and androstenedione (a steroid hormone that later produces estrogen or testosterone), the hormone that fuels sexual development.

The first menstruation is often a charged event for incest victims. Partly because of the confused dynamics in the family with borderline behaviors, many have been mocked, ridiculed by parents who have acted without limits by, for example, telling everyone in the family openly about the child's menstrual debut. Many patients testify that the first menstruation has either been exaggerated or completely downplayed/ignored by not receiving any guidance with menstrual protection or explanation of what is happening. Mothers who have known about the incest have sometimes openly shown disgust or envy that they are now an adult *partner* to the father. But it also means that the girl can have children, which changes the conditions for penetrative abuse, and that the pedophile's sexual preference can either be strengthened or ended at puberty. Cell changes are also common in incest survivors earlier than what healthcare calls their continuous Pap smear examinations, due to early penetrative abuse.

Dental health is also negatively affected for incest survivors. According to Walker et al., (1996); Willumsen et al., (2004); Stalker et al., (2005); Uziel et al., (2012); referenced in Wolf, McCarty & Priebe, (2020), victims of sexual violence experience more anxiety and worry than other patients during dental visits, such as perceived discomfort associated with instruments in the mouth, increased gag reflex, difficulty being quiet and relaxed, an aversion to being touched, and exaggerated feelings of loss of control. The study involved 11 women with experiences of childhood sexual abuse in relation to psychological and physical reactions to the dentist. An overarching theme was that the visit was like an echo of traumatic abuse from the past that resulted in dysfunctional reactions. They were reluctant to go to the dentist or canceled/did not show up to a higher extent than non-victims. They described a feeling of being locked in the dentist's chair, the horizontal inclination of the body was mentioned as a reason. Not telling about their previous experiences of sexual abuse was more the rule than the exception. They also did not mention their fear of the dentist. During the visit, respondents described dissociative reactions such as stopping breathing, freezing, becoming paralyzed and an inability to speak. One respondent described it as if in the event of sexual abuse as a child, one could only accept what happened and that she was put in the same state at the dentist. The visit reactivates high anxiety even though the real danger was over long ago. If they had told her that she needed to have all her teeth pulled, she would have just accepted it (trauma response fawn). For dentists and other staff, it is important to pay attention to whether the patient's gaze changed during the treatment (dissociation), a desire to rinse her mouth frequently, a constant flood of tears, cramps in the body and dizziness (Wolf, McCarty & Pribe, 2020).

When a child is exposed to constant painful and prolonged abuse that they have had to endure and dissociate in order to survive, they often have difficulty with normal pain sensations. For example, they may have difficulty determining whether the bath water is too hot or cold, when they have hurt themselves, tend to ignore fatigue, hunger and other bodily needs to the detriment of their physical well-being. Many times their bodies suffer from neglect in adulthood. But there may also be parts that are mute, hypersensitive to the slightest physical change and find even a low level of pain or discomfort unbearable (Boon, Steele & Van De Hart, 2012).

Complex post-traumatic stress disorder (CPTSD) and dissociative disorders are diagnoses that describe the severe traumatization that people can experience from war experiences and torture. However, the greatest risk factor for these disorders is repeated childhood sexual abuse, and more people are affected by CPTSD than by the simpler form PTSD.

In PTSD, it is a single extreme event that creates an uncontrolled and disabling re-experiencing of memories, emotions and thoughts from the extreme event. However, with access to the right treatment, it is possible to quickly regain a well-functioning life. The vast majority of patients with PTSD heal their injuries themselves and do not need specialist care.

In CPTSD, however, it is usually repeated extreme events during childhood that the child cannot escape that are the basis for the illness. Such as incest. The constant stress that children exposed to incest and other sexual abuse live with risks damaging brain development and creating imbalances in all of the body's systems as a result. CPTSD can therefore be seen as a systemic illness, and it often causes several different illnesses, both physical and mental, so-called comorbidity. The comorbidity is so serious that life expectancy can be shortened by up to 20 years, and the risk of suicide is high if curative treatment is not given.

A good exercise for victims of sexual violence is to ask them about a time when they listened to their body and acted on the information or did not act. Victims of sexual violence often need to learn to set boundaries and care for your own body. In healthcare, we need to make the patient aware of how much information the body actually gives you.

Treatment SAIS, 1-4 PTSD and CPTSD

There is a before and an after of the first time one enters the world through the eyes of a child who encounters indifference and evil. Trauma always involves a violation of the word no. A trauma memory differs from a person's biographical narrative memory because parts or all of the memory is dissociated (Boon, 2017). The treatment of patients who have been exposed to sexual abuse in childhood, incest and/or trafficking, organized and ritual sexual abuse therefore needs to be particularly person-centered based on where the patient is, respectful and responsive. Patients are found in all strata of society, in all healthcare settings, some are walking through life alone, others have beloved family members around them and some have people around them who are unable to bear the burden that incest and sexual abuse of children can entail. It can be unbearable for a relative to listen to details about when someone they love was intentionally harmed as a child, but even though it is difficult to listen, it is important to know that it is when the details emerge that the patient is set free. Unfortunately, the devil is often in the details. When the details are exposed, we can talk about the shame. Trauma means wound, which in turn comes from the word to pierce (Laplache & Pontalis, 1988). Synonyms for pierce are to penetrate, impale, nail, puncture, prick or wound. There are many words to describe the violation that has occurred of the patient's no. Which consequently leads to both pain and anger towards the perpetrator, other family members, organizations and society that failed to protect them as children.

Healthcare has a clear responsibility to detect and identify patients who are and have been exposed to violence and to provide adequate medical and psychosocial care. There is currently a lack of both care programs and guidelines for working with deep dissociative states after sexual violence. The boundary between psychiatric and somatic care after sexual violence overlaps and merges, both in the trauma itself, the symptoms and the care afterwards. This is problematic when a somatic intervention, for example, risks being psychologically harmful to the patient.

Patients at Wonsa and many more victims testify to clear shortcomings in treatment, treatment in the non-acute phase in particular. Accounts of lack of treatment or inappropriate treatment. Care that has been pointless or, in the worst case, harmful, with outright abuse. SOU (2023) provides sharp criticism regarding serious shortcomings within the regions and municipalities regarding help for sexually abused people in the non-acute phase. The shortcomings relate primarily to identification, knowledge of the vulnerability and treatment, access to non-acute care and trauma treatment, access to care outside metropolitan regions, and the division of responsibilities and coordination between the authorities. The voluntary organizations that meet the target groups confirm the shortcomings that their members experience.

There are several theories as to why sexual violence is not recognized in healthcare. Häggblom et al., (2005) show that the main reason why nurses in healthcare do not ask about the patient's previous sexual abuse is that they want to show respect for the woman's integrity. This is followed by the nurses experiencing difficulties in formulating the question and deficiencies in knowledge about handling abuse, fear of the answer and lack of time. Many describe feeling uncertain about where to refer the patient. We can only hope that the two specialist clinics that have now opened in Stockholm and Gothenburg will increase the courage of other agencies to ask about sexual abuse in the past and present. Now that there is a clinic to refer to. Another difficulty in detecting sexually abused patients can be expressed in terms of co-morbidity, the condition when one diagnosis is the basis for another diagnosis that sexual abuse generates. Which leads to the caregiver often missing the basic problem. The patient may be afraid to ask specific questions and the healthcare provider rarely investigates sexual violence, especially in non-acute stages. Treatment is therefore only focused on the obvious symptoms, such as antidepressants for depressive symptoms (Rayan, et al., 2017).

Transference and countertransference

Yalom (1989) talks about the therapist's responsibility to create a relationship where the patient needs to dare to understand, verbalize and face their inner demons in a trusting therapy relationship. But it is required that therapists are willing to explore using themselves as a tool. In the transference with severely traumatized patients, the therapist will, among other things, represent a savior, incompetent, useless, dangerous, controlling, evil, have a hidden agenda or be about to leave the patient. Which can lead to the therapist in the countertransference feeling that nothing I do is good enough, the patient is too demanding, she takes up all my energy and time, I can't stand this patient, it's a hopeless case or I'm a failed therapist. The countertransference can also lead to the therapist feeling that this patient has suffered so much that I have to do more than is recommended, in this particular situation I can give out my private phone number, it's completely fascinating to work with this patient or she will kill herself if I stop (Boon, 2017).

In relation to sexual abuse between adults in general, there are always gray areas, dividing lines that have been crossed when failed intercourse or rough sex turns into rape. It is not always prominent in the story or for the patient themselves. But when the line has been crossed, the therapist needs to demonstrate the law of consent and its limits through psychoeducation. Many young people come to me with multiple sexual experiences that are borderline or obvious rapes that they themselves are not aware of. Young people who believe that you have to put up with strangulation, group or anal sex if your partner wants it. As a therapist, it is also about choosing to understand without interpreting events that the patient has not experienced as borderline, but the therapist does. We have a task to be neutral and to the law of consent, but also to be open to patients giving consent to sexual acts that the therapist personally believes are borderline. The therapist's personal interpretations make the therapist who they are and thus become the starting point for which interventions the therapist chooses to make or not make. As psychotherapists, we bring our own countertransferences, tendencies, our history of relationships and our own traumas into the therapeutic relationship. In a study, Wickström (2016) investigated how psychotherapists deal with shame and argued that empathy, self-compassion and understanding of their own feelings of shame were required to be able to understand the patient in depth. The stronger our countertransference reactions are, the less fluent we are and the less able we are to work skillfully with our patients (Wolterstorff & Grassman, 2013).

According to Hahn (2004), shame often occurs in a negative therapeutic reaction. This can mean that when the white shame created by childhood sexual abuse is revealed, symptoms will worsen, progress will cease and feelings of inadequacy and hostility will arise in the countertransference. It takes courage to face the shame and accept it as a therapist; a vacuum will arise before we separate ourselves from the patient's shame and reach a state of our own freedom from shame. In our treatment, we must not turn a blind eye to the shame; we need to accept it, shelter it and process the anger and resentment that the patient carries. We need to carry the patient's anger until she is ready to take it back, but then in a melted form. The suffering after a lifetime of incest or sexual abuse can be experienced as unfair, merciless and unbearable. As psychotherapists and doctors, we often encounter suicidal patients where the death drive is constantly present and the pain is embodied in both body and soul. Early attachment relationships that have repeatedly failed in their emotional tone play a crucial role in how shame manifests itself in the adult patient. As a therapist, you may be held responsible for the patient's negative transference, which affects countertransference. Strong feelings of jealousy where the patient sometimes wants everything that you as a therapist can offer, which turns into envy and a desire to destroy the object (the therapist). As a therapist, you need to have the knowledge and tools to identify the patient's feelings of shame, otherwise the patient will feel misunderstood and end their therapy prematurely or lead to the problem remaining. Shame can also lead to the patient's empathy decreasing as self-focus increases, which can result in both aggressive and unfriendly behavior. The point here is to accommodate the patient's feelings and attacks both against you as a therapist and against the patient themselves without taking revenge or letting a feeling of being a useless therapist take over.

According to Kluft (2010), the patient often takes in other persecutory evil objects and transfers them onto the therapist. One needs to put up with the patient's insecure attachment patterns and sometimes have to represent the perpetrator in the transference. We intrude by showing that a close relationship is possible. The therapist's kindness and benevolence can be met with distrust or accusations and sometimes misunderstood by the patient as seductive motives. Even if the therapy goes well, the patient will wait for the therapist to show his true side and humiliate, exploit and abandon her. The patient may also fantasize that their own badness is contagious and can corrupt the therapist. The patient projects what is unbearable within themselves onto the therapist who in turn becomes a persecutory object. A large part of the treatment will be about the perception that the incest or sexual abuse is their own fault, especially in the case of multiple perpetrators where the patient can see no other explanation than that it is their own fault. Why else would so many choose to abuse them?

Subjective perspective

Wolterstorff & Grassman, (2013) propose a theory that traumatic memories of sexual abuse perpetrated by a family member such as incest, someone at school or church are more complex than traumatic memories of, for example, a car accident, surgery or being attacked by a stranger. Due to the nature of close relationships. To conceptualize "in-group" trauma where the perpetrator is someone close to the patient, the authors suggest that the patient needs to see themselves in the memory from four different roles; a) the rescuer, the victim, the bystander and the perpetrator, b) all roles can develop PTSD symptoms. Since trauma memories are subjective, all different roles have experienced different scenarios during a traumatic event. The rescuer may develop secondary traumatization, the rescuer and the bystander may develop survivor guilt from having observed the trauma. According to the authors, the most post-traumatic dysfunctions are found in the perpetrator, such as addiction, suicide and repetition compulsion, c) during a traumatic event we do not remember much of what happened to ourselves but rather a subjective interpretation of the entire traumatic incident, we remember the scene at the crime scene, d) in order to heal from a complex relational trauma, the patient needs to integrate all four post-traumatic roles and the entire traumatic event. By identifying with one role and not identifying with others as one usually does, the patient has a superficial misinterpretation of what actually happened. You remember what you think happened and what you think others present experienced. But the memory of the entire scene is there whether we want it or not. Like a director, the patient assigns roles in the traumatic scene and interacts with them as if they were actors on a stage. But a person can have more than one role, as trauma is often complex. The mother can be both the rescuer and the spectator. She has both sanctioned the incest by doing nothing for a period and later been the one who stopped it. The authors suggest that in order to heal, the patient in the therapy room needs to remember all roles correctly, to achieve symptom reduction, integrate the memory of all four roles, by playing all roles. The spectator needs to integrate the victim, the perpetrator needs to integrate experiences of the rescuer and finally the victim needs to integrate (previously imagined) experiences of the perpetrator. By seeing the perpetrator's situation and motives, the picture of the memory becomes more nuanced for the victim. Integrating does not mean feeling empathy, feeling empathy does not mean feeling sympathy or that it is an excuse to forgive. Instead, it leads the patient to consciously come to the realization that non-owned parts of our minds exert control over us until we have absorbed and digested it.

A safe place

According to Kluft (2010), there are few topics in the therapy room that confront the therapist with such complex, painful and potential clinical dilemmas as incest committed by a close family member. Wolterstorff & Grassman (2013) argue that psychotherapists have long argued that non-integrated traumatic events force us to revisit them, by re-entering the crime scene or through repetition compulsion. For the patient, the therapy room is a safe place with clear boundaries. Here they are allowed to visit traumatic memories together with the psychologist or psychotherapist. The stories can be fragmented, cut off at emotions or razor-sharp. The feelings are either dissociated or intact, moods and pain are experienced here and now. The body cannot distinguish between what happened to them a long time ago and what is happening right now. Past and present are intertwined.

Part of the treatment involves helping the patient create a safe and comfortable place where they can rest after we have visited their child self in vulnerable situations. The therapist's job is to lead the patient to a peaceful, comfortable and pleasant place, we go through the abuse together, move to a safe place and then back to the present. You are here and now, do you remember how it felt when you took the elevator up to the reception, when you sat in the waiting room and that everything we talked about today belongs to the past. It can no longer hurt you. It is completely over. We show the way from the past to the present. Together we have just walked through thorny blackberry thickets where the patient was dragged as a child, we are looking for a way out and the thorns grab us, tear open small wounds on the patient's body that dig under their child's skin. If the thorns are not taken out, the wounds will become inflamed and start to hurt. Our job as therapists is to look for the invisible thorns and gently pull them out one by one, until the skin and body are free from the abuser's violence. We go into the blackberry thicket together and we come out together.

In trauma treatment we build new safe rooms and places where the patient's child self can rest after they have come out of the blackberry thicket. Fantasy castles by the sea that are protected by all imaginable beings, God figures and legends we create, mountain cabins, huts and beach houses that exist on other planets or in a hot air balloon. Moats with water that no one can travel on because they are filled with crocodiles that keep the perpetrator outside, and the child inside its protective circle. Good monsters that work *with* the child, gives them back a sense of control and power that keeps other monsters away. We fantasize about armor that makes them invisible or has special force fields. After the treatment, the child self is allowed to move home to the patient where they live now, indefinitely. They never have to move back to the home they hate. In the first phase of therapy, we work to create welcoming safe places where the patient's child self can move when they have stepped out of the trauma period after the treatment. Below, a patient talks about her imagined safe place.

Villa Solviken

By patient Sindra, SAIS 6 DID - www.didyouknow.se

Did you know that there is a place, a place that is completely safe where no harm can reach you? I would like to tell you about life in Villa Vila at Solviken in Stilla Land. There is a place prepared where anyone who so wishes can move into the big white house on the peninsula by the lake in Solviken in Stilla Land. There My Father the King is waiting for you, the Good Shepherd Jesus Christ, the True Holy Spirit. You are welcome to move there with all parts of you and all those who want to help you. Come with me and we will see what the house looks like.

First we come to the big white wall. At the entrance there is a gate and there are two tall angels standing at the gate, letting in and letting out the helpers who are going to the place. When we enter the garden we are met by an avenue and on each side there is the most beautiful orchard you can imagine. Right now it is approaching autumn and then the garden looks the way it does when the garden is preparing for winter rest. Directly to the left is a small house, a small guardhouse. That is where all the helpers can go and unload their burdens and talk with my father the king.

Let's walk down the avenue to the entrance, the large round wooden staircase into the large white wooden house. An incredibly beautiful villa where the joy of carpentry has taken different forms and which can be transformed and rebuilt exactly as you want it in your story. To the right on the outside you can see a tower room. Your gaze will immediately be drawn there. There is something about the building that is strange, but at the same time beautiful. When you enter the house, you enter a waiting room. It is a rectangular-shaped waiting room with high windows on the left side out into the garden and straight ahead are two large white double doors. Everyone who comes to the house knows that only the people who live in the house are allowed to go in there. The helpers who come are allowed to go in and open the large white wooden doors into the large conversation room. There is so much light in this room. Immediately when you enter the room in the right corner there is a large open fireplace and the strange thing is that in that fireplace there is always a fire burning, just like now. You can hear the fire crackling. Along the far wall there is a corner sofa there from the corner the sofa runs out into the room. I usually sit in that corner. Maybe you will sit there one day? In front of the oxblood-colored sofa is a table. On the table is a worn old Family Bible. It is well read and it is often used in the morning hours by the fire. What you will be struck by is that on the beautiful wooden floor is a gigantic, large, round rug, a rug that is soft, thick and warm and has the image of a sunflower. On the sunflower rug my sisters and I usually have our morning meetings together with our helpers. Maybe you will also have meetings here one day? With whom I don't know, but you know that. By the window are two solid gray armchairs and between them is a small glass table. On that glass table you put important things. Right now, as you can see, there are a number of slides on the table. When they are against the glass, they are white frames with black squares inside, but I know and you know that every time I and one of my helpers choose to lift one of those pictures and choose to hold them up to the light, because you know in the Pacific, the sun shines most of the time and when we feel the warmth from the sun's rays, we know that it is the warmth both from the love of My Father the King, the light radiates from Him. He is the source of all life, light and warmth. Every time you lift a slide and let the light filter through, we know that it is God's truth that shines through the brutal, terrible events in our lives.

Behind one armchair and the wall is a large white screen. On the screen, sequences from my life, perhaps from your life, can be played, but the amazing thing is that in this conversation room everything is safe. It is in this place that my half-sisters and I share the truth about our lives, but we don't have to be afraid because there is always someone with us. I always have one of my helpers with me when I face the past. I am no longer alone, not alone with my thoughts, feelings, reactions. There is always someone there who can hold my hand, assure me that I am safe, that I have survived, that no one can hurt me or my half-sisters anymore. So in this place you can put down burdens. In this place you can also leave the heavy and difficult to go back into the house or out into the garden.

Let me tell you more about the house. When you come out of the waiting room and when you are trusted and allowed to go into the rest of the house, you come out into a hall and in that hall is the entrance to one of the most beautiful bathrooms you have ever seen, decorated in exactly the way you need. Straight ahead with windows facing the orchard is the large farmhouse-like kitchen and the strange thing about this room is that there is always a strong deep scent of freshly baked bread or buns. Don't ask me how it works, but it feels like Siv, who is the housekeeper and takes care of everything practical, always has a bun dough in the works. Both my half-sisters and I love being here because in this kitchen you can just sit. You don't have to say much, you get to participate in a warm community, just sit and think. It is also here that every evening everyone, at the same time, has an evening coffee with The Good Shepherd. You know the One who stands at the door and knocks, if anyone hears his voice, he is welcome in and you can have a meal together. So the Good Shepherd has said from the beginning, firmly and kindly: I want to talk to you all in the evening. I want to hear how your day has been and I am interested in everything, not just who you have talked to about God or what you have accomplished but how it has felt and how you have measured and how your thoughts are going, about small things and about big things. The conversation with the Good Shepherd every evening creates stability in everyday life.

But what happens in the mornings? Well, I'll tell you. If you walked into the house one morning and passed the kitchen on the right and came into the large dining room. There is the largest, white, oval wooden table you have ever seen with beautiful carved wooden chairs all around. To the left of the high seat always sits my Father the King. Maybe you will sit there one day? Then everyone in the house is around the table, all my half-sisters, from the youngest to the oldest. There is also Siv who participates in the meal and the fellowship. There is also Sanna, the Holy Spirit. There is also The Good Shepherd. It is a bit difficult. He smells a bit of a shepherd. It smells of sheep at every breakfast, but My Father the King sits in all his splendor on the high seat and his warm gaze meets each of our gazes. Maybe his gaze will meet yours one day? At breakfast we usually plan the day. What is going to happen today? Who is going to talk in the conversation room with one of the Helpers? Who will help the Good Shepherd take care of and bring the lambs into the large sheepfold that is on the slope behind the house down towards the lake? Who will help with the practical things in the garden? Yes, there is a lot to do, especially now that Christmas is approaching. There is an expectation in the air. Often it is the case that My Father the King decides to go out for a walk with one of the half-sisters or with me. Maybe he will take a walk with you in the future? That is up to you.

Let's go upstairs, which really only consists of two things. When you come up the big wooden staircase that faces the lake with big windows, there's my big studio and on the big, old, slightly worn wooden floor lies a gigantic rag rug. The rag rug of life.

I know that the walls will be filled with paintings – paintings where each of my half-sisters expresses their story. Where each of my half-sisters has the opportunity to give their image of the secret that they have carried and that they have carried for me throughout their lives. To the right and with a lot of air around there is a large white grand piano, where I sit and compose. I have created a lot of music in this time since I moved into the house.

Wall to wall with my studio is a large, bright nursery that is arranged like a fan where each of my smaller half-sisters has their own space that is decorated just the way they need it. In this room there is also space for shared play and games and fellowship. There is also a staircase up to a loft, to the tower room. The tower room that is currently being decorated for one of the smallest.

Now that you have seen the inside of the house, let's go outside and see what the garden looks like. If you follow the path along Solviken and over to the right, on the right side of the lake, there is a small convent. I am the abbess of that convent. I am the one who decides there too.

On the left side of the lake, quite far away so that it is almost impossible to see, at least not if you see as little as I do, there lies the Village of the Forgotten and the Chosen. There, in a band of boathouses along the water's edge, tastefully and personally decorated, lives every person I love and who also needs companionship with this fantastic trio that I have mentioned. They live there and the beautiful thing is that even if they feel alone, forgotten, perhaps not seen, they are because they are chosen. They were already that when they were in their mother's womb and the care from the heavenly trio – the Father, the Son, the Spirit – is total. I have finally managed to let go and can concentrate on life in Villa Vila.

Now you have heard a little more about life in Villa Vila at Solviken in Stilla Land. A place that I have co-created together with my helpers and together with Sanna, the Holy Spirit, a place that is safe. A place where I can find rest right now. A place where I can heal. When the pain, sadness, anger and fear have been safely allowed to come out into the conversation room and when each half-sister's story has been translated into colors and come up along the walls of the conversation room. Then it is time for me to return to the Land of Suffering or yes, the true description is probably the Land of Hope and Suffering, then this place is ready to receive you and your inner family, what you are thinking of. The beautiful thing about it all is that you don't have to wait to move in until I am finished with my process. This place is always prepared for you. I want to continue sharing my story with you because I believe it can give you hope and comfort where you are, but today, remember the last impression I want to leave on your retina. That is, if you look down towards the shore, you can see the eternal, sacred ring dance. If you look down towards the water, you see My Father the King hand in hand with The Good Shepherd Jesus Christ and the True Holy Spirit, how in a single, eternal movement of love they have fellowship, honor each other and how they want to help the person who wants to come into the center of their fellowship and be marinated in the love that sustains the entire universe. This place is not just for me. It is also for you.

The relationship to anger

People who have been severely traumatized by others often experience strong feelings of anger, rage, hatred, and revenge. One of the most difficult aspects of anger and rage is its intense and overwhelmingly powerful physical sensation. Their anger at wrongs done to them is perfectly legitimate. Many patients experience a total fear of becoming angry, losing control, becoming like the perpetrator as an identification with the aggressor. When anger and rage are not directed outward, but inward, they are often transformed into suicidal thoughts, self-harm, or chronic self-loathing (Boon, Steele, Van Der Hart, 2012). Greenfield (2012) describes a seven-year psychodynamic therapy with a 55-year-old woman who was chronically suicidal. She was raised by a sadistic and narcissistic mother and a father who sexually abused her between the ages of 6 and 9. At times, her suffering and imminent desire to commit suicide could arouse existential uncertainty in the therapist's own role. A whispering voice within the therapist said why is he prolonging her suffering by continuing to keep her alive. The therapy room is an oasis of projections, older haunting objects, absent good objects, transference and countertransference. It is especially difficult when the patient's perpetrator is the mother. Among boys who have been subjected to incest by their mother, according to family therapist Haliburn, (2017); referenced in Johansson & Svedin, (2021) it is most typical that during the abuse they felt very special and chosen and that they did not see their physical relationship with the mother as sexual abuse but more as a relationship. Haliburn states that sexual abuse committed by the mother leaves lasting harm and deep wounds within the patient that affect the child's self-esteem and relationships later in life.

Tolerance window

It is difficult to treat patients with multiple childhood sexual abuse. Often the patient comes in with multiple diagnoses, a broad symptom picture and dissociated memories. Boon, Steele & Van Der Hart (2012) believe that diagnoses are not labels that tell who the patient is but rather a way to categorize a spectrum of different experiences. The therapeutic framework is central to every agreement on psychotherapy. Concepts such as the therapy being non-evaluative, non-judgmental and non-positional distinguish an analytic conversation from an everyday conversation (Gullestad & Killingmo, 2005). An important task in all psychotherapy, but especially trauma treatment, is that the patient is at an optimal level of tension, the so-called tolerance window. Each of us has an individual tolerance level that is to some extent determined by our innate temperament and our physiological reactions. But it is also determined by our experiences, when we have been flooded with affects for a long time, our ability to regulate affect will eventually become overloaded (Van der Hart et al., 2006). The Window of Tolerance is Dan Siegel's model for understanding how our nervous system reacts to stress both emotionally and physiologically. When the patient is in the tolerance window, they are in a state where they can feel, think and act in a flexible, adaptive way without being overwhelmed. When anxiety increases or triggers some trauma, the patient can step out of the window. This can happen via hyperarousal (overactivation), the patient becomes anxious, restless, angry, has panic attacks, physical symptoms of anxiety as the sympathetic nervous system accelerates by preparing the body for fight or flight. If the patient falls below the tolerance window, they will fall into hypoarousal (underactivation) which leads to withdrawal. Here the patient may feel empty, numb, indifferent or experience their body as heavy and sunken. A kind of freeze or collapse that is often linked to a feeling of powerlessness. The tolerance window is not a fixed zone but a dynamic range. Siegal talks about the body having a baseline, a calibrated window to which it always returns.

Resilience

It is often said that life does not come with a map, resilience is the process or ability to successfully adapt to difficult or challenging life experiences. Which means that an individual has mental, emotional and behavioral flexibility and adaptability to external as well as internal changes. How a person sees their world and engages in it, access to social resources and specific coping strategies are important factors in how well we adapt to new conditions. Our existence will involve challenges for everyone, it is part of our human condition. The word survivor or dandelion child is the correct term for incest survivors and survivors of ritual and organized sexual abuse of children, which shows the essence of resilience, we can move on, despite unbearable experiences. In working with the target group, the concept of resilience becomes leading and we understand why it is dandelions that light up the summer meadows and can grow through the asphalt. When researchers Hellman & Mattis (2023) are interviewed about why it is important to feel and convey hope in the therapy room, they believe that hope is not an unrealistic luxury but a necessary experience. Being hopeful about the future is necessary to move forward after trauma. In the book Hope rising: How the Science of Hope Can Change Your Life, Hellman defines the phenomenon of hope as the belief that tomorrow can be better than today and that we have the ability and agency to change our situation. Hope is a verb, it is something we do. Which means that hope is a cognitive process, something we think about rather than a feeling. The difference between hope and optimism is that the optimistic person has an expectation that something will go well, while the hopeful person has an expectation and a plan. When you have lost hope, you do not see any way to influence your situation, which in turn increases the risk of becoming suicidal. Traumatic events in childhood rob us of hope to some extent, especially early traumas, here hopefulness needs to be allowed to creep in during the course of treatment. But in the meantime, the therapist needs to act as a substitute hope until the patient is able to set their own goals for a better tomorrow.

Forgiveness

Forgiveness is not the first thing that comes to mind when dealing with survivors of incest and child sexual abuse. According to Enright, Eastin, Golden Sarinopulous & Freedman, (1992); referenced in Freedman, (1999), the concept of forgiveness is often misunderstood, especially in relation to survivors of incest. The definition of forgiveness involves letting go of resentment/bitterness, which leads to letting go of the harm that could occur if one were to retaliate. Our feelings, thoughts and behavior change in a positive direction when we go through the forgiveness process Augsburger, (1970); Droll, (1984); Smedes, (1984); referenced in Freedman, (1999).

Olio, (1992); referenced in Freedman, (1999) argues that forgiving interventions in the therapy room with incest survivors may risk leading to denial of the abuse or validation of the actions they were subjected to. It is therefore important to emphasize that forgiveness does not mean excusing, tolerating, forgetting or reducing one's angry feelings over time. In addition, we need to distinguish between forgiveness and reconciliation as two separate processes. We can forgive without being reconciled, but in order to be reconciled, the perpetrator's behavior needs to change Enright et al., (1991); Holmgren, (1993), Meek & McMinn, (1997); referenced in Freedman, (1999), that the perpetrator acknowledges his guilt. But only 1% of all convictions in sexual crime cases in Sweden are due to the perpetrator admitting the crime, which means that 99% deny it, reconciliation between perpetrator and victim is therefore unusual. As Lundberg (2023) states in her book, she can accept the childhood she had but she will never forgive her parents, as they lack remorse. According to Cotroneo, (1982); Hunter, (1979); Kaufman, (1989); referenced in Freedman & Enright, (1996), many clinical case studies show that anger, depression and anxiety are reduced when the victim has forgiven her perpetrator. Within psychodynamic therapy, there is a common thread of reconciliation and reparation. As psychotherapists, we almost always move towards reparation because of its healing power, except when working with incest. Incest is like no other crime. Forgiving can also be difficult to think about for the other parent, who did not commit the offense. According to Svedin and Banck (2002), the support that the child can receive from the non-offending parent is an important positive factor. A capable adult, if the abuse is discovered early, means that the child is more likely to develop positive adaptation strategies. However, processing becomes more difficult despite such care if there is a close relationship with the abuser (Tidefors Andersson, 2002).

Spirituality

It is important that as a therapist for severely traumatized individuals, one has an openness to the patient's relationship to spirituality. We need to be prepared for spiritual perspectives to emerge through the treatment that need to be included. The spiritual perspectives can be in conflict with our conventional Western view of consciousness and the relationship to body and mind. Alternative spiritual perspectives can challenge the therapist's own belief system and can sometimes be difficult to interpret. The therapist does not need to understand or have an opinion about the patient's experiences but needs to accept them as real and important aspects of the patient's healing process. In MDMA (central stimulant and hallucinogenic substance) assisted trauma therapy, the therapist should help the patient integrate spiritual experiences into daily life. These experiences can help the patient with a perspective that is not about their identification with their trauma, but a larger perspective on how they feel about themselves. Through their spirituality, they can become aware of their inner strength in order to thereby be able to integrate their traumatic experiences and move on in life.

Organization, work environment and self-care

Therapists and clinicians working with sexual violence need to developa certain tolerance and capacity to receive stories, never against the nature of the crime as such but as a therapist. Working with patients exposed to severe trauma is demanding, both for the patient and the staff. That the organization can provide both the patient and the staff with the support needed is important for a safe, sustainable and healing environment to be created. My experience is that the therapist himself, in addition to formal competence, knowledge and supervision, also needs to have his own inner security and knowledge of any dissociative injuries. It is difficult to help another across water that you yourself have not sailed, and it can easily become a trigger if you have not healed your own wounds. However, if you are prepared to do so as the challenges arise, working with traumatized patients offers lifelong personal development. In a study by Mentzer, Rembeck, Dahlberg, Premberg (2024), they interviewed (*N*=11) trauma therapists in Sweden who describe what it is like to be exposed to stories of torture, rape and to work with young and vulnerable individuals living in poverty and severe vulnerability, as well as working with cases of ongoing abuse and violence. These aspects were experienced by the respondents as the most difficult and challenging professional shields for therapists. Working with DID patients involves a difficulty in understanding and being able to relate as a non-traumatized person. We cannot understand DID patients by relating to something within ourselves as we usually can. We have all had a part of us that wants to go to a party and a part that wants to stay home, but that does not mean that we understand how the parts of a DID patient feel.

Dyregrov & Mitchell, (1992); Pearlman & Maclan, (1995)Tedeschi & Calhoun, (2004); Yassen, (1995); referenced in Mentzer et al., (2024) also mention that clinicians can have several positive effects from working with traumatized patients. Having the opportunity to help vulnerable individuals can contribute to better quality of life, personal relationships, personal strength and feelings of meaning. In Sweden, there are very few clinicians who are trained specialists in sexual violence against children, despite the high prevalence in our society. Almost all support and group activities that are conducted are carried out within civil society voluntary organizations by unlicensed personnel. We have a society that has handed over a large part of the responsibility to survivors who are supposed to help other survivors. The healthcare system has pointed out limitations regarding trauma therapy and few specialists in sexual abuse in a non-acute stage.

Lifespan Integration

Lifespan integration is a psychotherapeutic method that aims to help the body and brain heal after difficult experiences by integrating traumatic memories into the story of life. The method is both a gentle and profound form of treatment used to help patients with PTSD. Rajan et al., (2020) describe that sexual abuse has devastating health consequences but can be treated and healed. In a study, 24 women with PTSD symptoms received a modified Lifespan Integration (MLI) treatment of 90–140 minutes and a follow-up conversation. Of those who participated in the study, 72% had such a significant reduction in their PTSD symptoms that they were no longer considered to have PTSD, compared to 6% who did not receive any treatment. Lifespan integration (LI) is a gentle therapeutic method that enables rapid healing for people who have experienced painful and frightening experiences, including neglect and sexual abuse. The method works without re-traumatizing and is based on the inherent human ability to heal. LI is based on the therapist and the patient creating a timeline of memories from the patient's life. By guiding the patient along the timeline of memories from childhood to the present, the brain receives evidence that time has passed and the event is over. By redirecting the neural networks and integrating difficult events into the course of life, the patient gains access to their entire adult self and acts more age-appropriately in situations that were previously dysfunctional. The therapist then guides the patient through the imagination to a traumatic memory and provides what is needed to resolve the situation. LI is a gentle method that does not require the patient to relive the trauma in detail, which makes it particularly suitable for those who risk being overwhelmed by going into the details of the trauma. The method works particularly well with incest, which often consists of hundreds of often quite repetitive rapes, as it treats several memories within one treatment, which are similar to each other. Through suggestion, the memory is rewritten or overwritten and the patient receives symptom relief from PTSD symptoms linked to the memory that has been treated. After treatment, the patient may experience a reduction in their PTSD symptoms, improved self-esteem, a more age-appropriate response pattern to stressful situations, and an increased ability to appreciate relationships. The results are persistent and quality of life continues to improve over time after the potential traumatic event has been integrated (Lifespan Integration, 2025).

Group therapy

Gul et al., (2020) describe four stages that an incest survivor goes through to fully integrate what they have experienced. The first stage involves intrusive memories and other memories of the abuse beginning to come to mind. Several behavioral and psychological symptoms arise and here the incest is often still a secret and the victim blames herself for not doing anything. In the second stage, the victim begins to examine the meaning of the abuse, gains new insight into what incest means and its consequences. They gain an increased understanding of family dynamics and the motivation of the perpetrator. In the third stage, the victim begins to tackle the symptoms of the abuse. Here, the victim often seeks out discussion groups or treatment through healthcare. In the fourth stage, the victim begins to take back control of their own life and actively work towards a healthy life. Herman (1992) talks in the book *Trauma and recovery* it is argued that groups for survivors of incest can be a powerful source of affirmation and support, with the important element that the group maintains its main task of creating a safe and secure place to share and listen to others. It should be knowledge-oriented and educational, not exploratory. Meeting in a group is a proven effective form of therapy for survivors of incest. Wolterstorff & Grassman, (2013) refer to group therapy in relation to the psychodynamic literature and various techniques that are described. They recommend group leaders who are competent, approved by specialists for the assignment, and receive supervision as the work with trauma patients includes transference and countertransference. Working as a group leader requires adequate technical skills, self-awareness, mindfulness and humility in order not to risk retraumatizing the patients. When new elements emerge, participants can gain insight into factors that they were not previously aware of. First, the participant needs to create their own meaning structure of the story before the group and the group leader come up with questions and interpretations. Johansson & Svedin (2021) also address that groups should be divided into those with female and male perpetrators as there is a clear stigma surrounding female perpetrators.

According to Yang, Luo, Liu and Wang (2024), the use of social support when treating psychological problems has been confirmed in several studies. Therefore, it is valuable if DID patients, after they have achieved a certain stability in phase one of their therapy, should receive group therapy. The advantages of psychotherapeutic group therapy are that it includes the feeling of feeling separated, which is common for patients with DID. It also gives the patient an opportunity to interact with people of different genders and exchange secrets, as well as face feelings of loneliness in the more open climate of the group. Group therapy also gives the patient the opportunity to learn from each other and understand the sub-self more objectively, and gives them hope for recovery since different group members are at different stages of the therapy process.

Documentation

When keeping records or conducting investigations, descriptive words need to be used where it is clear who had the agency, what type of abuse the victim was subjected to and who the perpetrator is. We need to train ourselves in record keeping so that sexual abuse based on the SAIS degree is recorded and made clear to the reader. This is of particular importance if the patient chooses to report to the police, but above all to confirm to the patient that we have listened to and believed their story. The patient may not choose to report to the police today, but later in life, then the journal entries may be the only evidence. Write what is actually said in the therapy room in the words the patient used, do not rewrite, summarize, minimize or distort. The perpetrator's responsibility tends to be reduced by descriptions of his overwhelming feelings that could not be accommodated. Consider whether the perpetrator's emotional expressions belong in the victim's record. By describing that he was jealous or insane weare covering up the realization that he had an intention to use violence. Words like he *hit* her or knocked *her down* are not detailed enough to clarify what actually happened. By writing that every time he hit her he felt terribly guilty, we diminish the victim's experience. An alternative description is that every time he hit her she experienced fear and terrible pain. By describing the perpetrator's feelings and emotional pain, we displace the victim's (Wade, 2010). We can think about linguist Paul Grice's principles when we write journal: a) Quality: tell the truth, have evidence for what you say, b) Quantity: tell "just enough", neither too short nor too long-winded, c) Relevance: do not stray from the topic into irrelevant matters, d) Comprehension (manner): express yourself clearly and distinctly.

Journal entry woman SAIS 5 DID

The patient seeks medical attention for pain due to previous fractures, and during a doctor's visit she opens up about the ritual sexual abuse she was subjected to as a child. The female doctor replies - why are you telling me this? I am not a psychologist. The medical record afterwards only mentions the somatic problem and the doctor does not want to connect the damage the patient suffered through the abuse, such as broken ribs, to the sexual abuse.

Active defenses in survivors

We all develop and have access to defenses against anxiety to cope with our reality in which we live. Since incest and sexual abuse in childhood means a great strain on the emotional life of a child, strong, intact, impenetrable defenses need to be created. The psychological defenses are vital for the child who is exposed but often mean great suffering for the adult patient. Since the defenses are added in childhood but are carried throughout life. The psychological defenses are simply impractical and not age-appropriate for the adult patient to be able to live a full adult and emotional life. The child has adapted to survive abuse but it means difficulties in adapting to other parts of life. Anxiety is a strong reaction from the part of the nervous system that we cannot control, a fear or worry that is felt in the body. Physical symptoms such as diffuse and nagging anxiety, heart palpitations, rapid breathing, chest tightness, panic attacks or other bodily reactions. As humans, we do everything we can to escape anxiety because of its discomfort.

A basic rule is that it is people, places or situations that trigger the patient's anxiety. Boon, Steele and Van der Hart (2012) describe different types of triggers that arouse particularly high anxiety in survivors of incest and childhood sexual abuse; 1) Time-related triggers, for example, can be an anniversary reaction. For incest victims, all holidays are usually a reminder of the deviant family, which arouses high anxiety and saintly melancholy. 2) Place-related triggers, involve places where the abuse occurred that the patient actively avoids; for patients who have sold sex for money, the entire city may be mined. Many choose a therapist based on where in the city they have their clinic. Even places such as crowded waiting rooms, shopping malls, and grocery stores can arouse anxiety. 3) Relational triggers, come from the fact that many have rightly felt criticized, lonely, abandoned and misunderstood as children, which in adulthood can mean similar feelings in relationships. Close relationships, where you need to trust someone, become especially revealing and vulnerable, you go and wait, looking for hints that you will be rejected or criticized. 4) Internal triggers, when internal experiences such as sensory sensations of pain or anxiety, anger or shame trigger. How someone speaks to us, loud noises, screaming or when someone shows emotions. 5) Sensory triggers, involve bodily sensations of, for example, smells, pain, heart palpitations or difficulty breathing. If you feel cold, hot, nauseous, thirsty, need to go to the toilet or during menstruation. But above all sensory memories that are brought to life by being touched on the body by others.

We have many defenses against anxiety, the more defenses a person has access to, the more well-functioning they are. We divide the defenses into two groups, the primitive primary defense processes that we usually talk about as the psychotic defenses and the secondary, more developed defense processes that we can think of as the neurotic defenses. McWilliams (2011) names the primitive defenses; primitive withdrawal, denial, omnipotent control, primitive idealization, primitive devaluation, projection, projective identification, splitting and dissociation. The more developed defenses are; repression, regression, isolation, intellectualization, rationalization, moralization, incoherence, annulment, turning towards the self, displacement, reaction formation, reversal into opposite, acting out, sexualization and sublimation.

Few available defenses lead to rigidity and monotonous ways of dealing with their life and anxiety. We can sort out the defenses that the child uses to survive the sexual abuse in the moment, between the abuse and afterwards, and to cope with their everyday life as an adult.

Denial

SAIS grade 1-3

Denial is often an active defense when the abuse is taking place, but can also be used after the abuse to protect oneself from the high anxiety that knowledge would generate. One denies what happened. For the small child, it is a way of dealing with unpleasant experiences by refusing to accept that it happened. We use denial in order to make life less unpleasant. In war, people have performed heroic actions by keeping *a cool head* in terrible and life-threatening situations. But the defense can also be used negatively by denying symptoms of an illness and not going to see a doctor. Many incest survivors testify about mothers who denied important signals from the child who is being abused, or that they denied that someone close to them could be an abuser. Tener et al., (2018) claim that the most common form of sexual abuse within the family is when one sibling abuses another sibling. When this happens, the most common attitude on the part of parents is that they deny that it happened. Bowlby (1980); referenced in Shaken, Benismon & Mashiach, (2021) believes that when a parent denies that the sexual abuse is taking place at the same time as it is happening, a conflict is created within the child with two separate models of reality. In order to reconcile the parents' denial with the abuse, the child accepts the parent's reality because challenging the parent may be associated with threats and tangible punishment. Survivors of incest who choose to inform relatives or report the crime to the police often receive negative reactions ranging from total denial, to being accused of the abuse themselves, to being expected to forgive the perpetrator Kennedy, (2000); Lamb & Edgar-Smith, (1994); referenced in Shaked, Benismon & Mashiach, (2021).

Journal entry woman SAIS 4

The patient expresses fear of being seen as a frivolous swindler without a basis in reality, as her family has tried to have her declared a minor.

Primitive withdrawal

SAIS grade 2-4

The defense of withdrawal is common in sexually abused children. It can involve the child withdrawing emotionally or psychologically, and can be experienced as entering a different state of experience or feeling. Physically, it means that the child withdraws from social situations or relationships and this is often replaced with their own internal simulated world or getting stuck in the digital world. A tendency to use drugs to reach a different state of consciousness can be considered a withdrawal. Withdrawal involves a certain psychological *escape* from reality but rarely a distortion of it. Here, one relieves one's anxiety by avoiding the world, not by misunderstanding it. One is aware of what is happening and what one is exposed to, but the child escapes into the world of games, the mobile phone or oneself. Many victims of incest describe that they built their own worlds where no one could reach them. It was both a way of escaping into oneself and a way of keeping the perpetrator outside.

Projecting

SAIS grade 2-5

Children and teenagers cannot stand their anxiety and an effective way to reduce or get rid of it is to project it onto someone else. What is unpleasant within me I attribute to you. Some children become overactive and projection is usually described as a defense where the psychological boundary between the self and the outside world is missing. *I feel bad and it's your fault,* it becomes difficult to distinguish between me and the outside world. A projection is when something that is inside me becomes wrongfully interpreted as being believed to come from the outside. In its healthy form, this is empathy. I feel bad when I hear your story. People in love can read each other's minds in a way that cannot be explained logically. They unconsciously project onto each other. You and I become one we.

Patients often testify about perpetrators who have projected their own agency and desire onto the child. The projections attributed to the child often lead to shame, guilt and feelings of disgust. In the therapy room, the patient needs help distinguishing between the projections from the perpetrator and what they themselves really felt. To the recipient, projections can feel like the sticky, stretchy, rubber hands of toys, they are thrown and get stuck and etched. Confusion arises when the child actually experienced powerful pain, discomfort and fear during the abuse while the perpetrator has attributed agency, arousal and pleasure to them. Vulnerable children may also use projection towards younger siblings or other children and subject them to violence or abuse.

Journal entry woman SAIS 4

She describes her ex-partner as very kind and feels sympathy for him because he is always remorseful after the rapes. She medicated with drugs and sleeping pills and woke up to find him raping her. He attributed the agency to her by saying I can see you want this.

Turning towards the self

SAIS grade 2-5

Children cannot choose their parents, nor can they understand that how their parents act towards them has nothing to do with them. Children believe until adolescence that everything that happens to them can be influenced by me and that it is my fault. They have no choice but to organize their world based on the one they actually live in in order to survive. Children who live in a horror movie under unbearable circumstances experience a total sense of loss of control. In order to regain some of the control that has been lost, the child will direct negative affects from the environment to the self. The child redirects criticism from the other to themselves. In this way, the child will experience that they can influence their environment. It is my fault that Dad is attacking me, there is something wrong with me, I am the one who is disgusting, that is why it happened to me, I have made him angry and need to be punished. As unpleasant as self-criticism may feel, it may be preferable to feeling threatened for life without having any power to change the situation. Defense often leads to self-hatred, one hates one's child self, which is experienced as disgusting, evil and seductive.

The child experiences the turning towards the self as more effective than the frightening alternative of survival being in the hands of an unreliable adult. This often leads to self-harming behaviour. Turning towards the self is a well-functioning defence for the small child but causes immense suffering for the adult patient. Children are programmed to be fundamentally loyal to their parents even if they are abusing them. Unlike adults, children have no one else to turn to. Many incest survivors describe hating their home. The terror and fear increase the need for attachment, even if the source of security was the same as the source of the fear. Summit (1983) describes it as if the attachment system and the fear system are intertwined, leading the child to believe that she caused the incest. In order to ensure her own survival, the child is unable to see the parent who abuses her as an evil object. Instead, the child sees the parent as good enough to ensure their survival. He calls this system a psychic economy, the child builds pockets of survival where the hope of goodness can live.

Sexualisation

SAIS grades 1-6

Sexualization can be seen as a form of acting out and is a human drive. Being sexually aroused is often associated with feeling alive. People have a tendency to eroticize people who possess power or celebrity and it is often a straightforward and harmless defense that we all use. However, when one has been subjected to sexual abuse, it can become a traumatic sexualization that leads to sexual exploitation or sex as self-harm. Children who have been subjected to sexual abuse by a father figure are always in a dependent position. Perpetrators use various ways to silence the child and a common way is to give the child positive attention or gifts. This can lead to traumatic sexualization, connecting abuse with positive reinforcement. Many incest survivors describe that the only time they received closeness and tenderness from their father was during an abuse. According to Donalek (2001), this can lead to the child learning to manipulate and use their sexuality as currency. Cabage et al., (2013) believe that children who have been sexually abused by their father experience that love involves sexual acts. Rathsman (2001) describes that girls can experience themselves as chosen and their father's confidant. It is as if the father and the girl speak their own language, have secrets, their own signals and signs that no one else can understand. Being chosen over her siblings and perhaps favored in social contexts by the father can make the girl feel complicit in the incest. Continuous threats, blaming, punishments and gifts lead to the girl not telling about the abuse. It is important to remember that the father figure is always the authoritarian in the relationship and controls it uninhibitedly. The fear of consequences that may arise if they tell is often total, the father threatens that the parents will separate, the family will suffer shame or that the father will end up in prison. In Nyberg and Dareflod's study from (2010), some of the respondents described that they discovered early on that they could get an exchange for sexual services and demand money or other things from the perpetrators. This exacerbated the feeling of shame, of being dirty and disgusting. According to Svedin and Banck (2002), it is common for vulnerable children to have an earlier sexual debut and other sexually risky behaviors. They bring up a teenage pregnancy as something to focus on. The sexual behavior problem can also be expressed through aggression, compulsive masturbation, a distorted perception of where the boundaries are or a wait-and-see behavior regarding sex. Children who have experienced sexual abuse have an increased risk of exposing another person to sexual abuse or being sexually abused by other perpetrators themselves.

Sex for money

SAIS grades 1-6

Children who have been exposed to incest are at increased risk of ending up in sexual exploitation and the path to this often goes through grooming, according to reports from the Swedish Agency for Gender Equality and the Swedish Children's Home (2021). Grooming usually takes place online and many are drawn into it via social media, dating sites, games or other digital forums for children and young people. Children have difficulty assessing risk and part of the grooming process involves the perpetrator finding ways to make themselves important in the child's life and building trust. Another path into sexual exploitation is through so-called sugar dating, which involves an older person, usually a man, giving some form of compensation for dating a younger person. According to research, previous sexual abuse in life is a well-known risk factor that can lead to a young person starting to receive compensation for sex. According to Jonsson & Svedin, (2015); referenced in SOU, (2023) it is a complex web of different factors that interact when young people begin to receive compensation for sex such as previous traumatic events, a feeling of being different and excluded. Svedin & Priebe, (2004); referenced in SOU, (2023) believe that sex for compensation for the young person is a way to feel seen, deal with traumatic events and regulate their emotions. In the Swedish Youth Agency's study from 2020/2021, a very high proportion of girls (88%) who received compensation for sex had been subjected to sexual abuse earlier in life compared to boys (36%). Knowledge about male sexual exploitation is more limited. In a survey from (2011) with (n=5071), the results showed that the men had several traumatic experiences in their lives such as being subjected to sexual acts by an adult outside the family, being subjected to violence in the family or having been subjected to violence or witnessed violence Jämställdhetsmyndigheten, (2021); referenced in SOU; (2023). In Gothenburg, it has been noted that gang criminal individuals sell women and young girls to each other for sexual exploitation, as a means of payment or as repayment of a debt. Many of them have previous experience of sexual abuse (Dagens Nyheter, 2023).

Sex as self-harm

SAIS grades 1-6

In psychiatry, various self-harm behaviors are a diagnostic criterion for EIPS (emotionally unstable personality disorder, previously called borderline personality syndrome), but are also found in other patient groups Bjärehed & Bjureberg, (2019); Cipriano, Cella & Cortrufo, (2017); referenced in Eriksson, (2022). The American Psychiatric Association, (2023) defines the concept of non-suicidal self injury (NSSI) and proposed criteria have been developed, as it is not yet seen as a diagnosis. Self-harm is when a person inflicts bodily harm that results in tissue damage, such as cutting, scratching, biting, rubbing the skin, self-starving, abusing drugs, burning, hitting or tearing open wounds. Research defines NSSI as; intentional actions, are directly directed at the person themselves, damage the body's tissues, are not carried out with suicidal intent and are not socially sanctioned or accepted. Indirect self-harm behaviors, such as self-destructive sex and substance abuse, are included in this definition (Nock, 2009). In Pettersson's (2013) study, respondents describe that they lost control of their bodies to the perpetrator during the sexual assault. This meant that later in life they experienced it as if they were regaining control over their lives by refusing food, harming themselves, abusing drugs or alcohol. Eriksson (2015) states that suffering leads to the individual tormenting themselves but can also include wanting to fight or endure. Several of my patients with an incest background who sell sex for money testify that they chose not to get drunk or take drugs before selling themselves in order to feel as much as possible. Klonsky, (2009); referenced in Zetterqvist, (2014) believes that the individual harms themselves to remove a feeling of emptiness, to feel numb and alone or to feel nothing at all. The research refers to self-destructive sex or sex as self-harm as a phenomenon, it lacks systematized knowledge and accepted conceptual conventions. According to Johan Bjureberg at the Karolinska Institute, young people experience that in the short term they can take control of their well-being by cutting themselves or through addiction, gambling, food or sex. He describes the role of the internet as both good and less good, positive that self-harm behaviors are highlighted so that knowledge increases but less good when there are so-called inspiration accounts, where social media shows pictures of wounds that can encourage the behavior. Another concern among researchers is that the internet makes it possible for young people to compete in who can hurt themselves the worst and thus increases the risk when the behavior escalates (SvD, 2018).

In the study Young, sex och internet from Linköping University (2014), it emerged that the group that used sex as self-harm showed the most trauma symptoms and felt the worst in relation to other groups that were subjected to abuse or sold sexual acts. According to Nina Rung, investigator at Barnahus (Stockholm Police), the target group is met with skepticism in psychiatry, healthcare and the legal system. She describes that when their cases end up with the Police, usually through the care of others, they are questioned and distrusted since they themselves were the ones who arranged to meet the men. Men who they know will harm them both physically and psychologically by using violence and humiliation in connection with sexual acts. One pattern is that the individual themselves seeks out destructive sexual situations or relationships, we can think of prostitution as a developed sexual self-harm behavior. An analogy could be that it is as if someone else is cutting your arms. But sex as self-harm leaves no visible scars or bruises on the body, only mental ones. With sex as self-harm, the individual has an increased loss of control as one or more perpetrators are included who influence the degree of harm inflicted, when you cut yourself, it is you who holds the object and controls the force of the self-harm behavior. In a Swedish study by Fredlund & Johansson, (2022); referenced in SOU, (2023) examined what people who had been sexually exploited and had sex as self-harm found to be helpful support. The study included 197 participants, mostly women with an average age of 27.9 years. The results showed three main themes about what the participants considered to be helpful as support for sex as self-harm; a) giving a word for the phenomenon (sex as self-harm), understanding that it exists and receiving questions and information about sex as self-harm and its function, b) flexible, respectful and professional help and support from an early age, being listened to and confirmed in their experience of sex as self-harm, and c) help with underlying causes in order to be able to get out of their self-harm. Finding one's self-worth and learning to set boundaries, through conventional therapy, through life itself and through therapy for underlying causes such as previous traumatic events, PTSD, dissociation or anxiety.

Journal entry woman SAIS 4

If an attractive man wants to have sex with me, it means I have value.

Journal entry woman SAIS 6 DID
The patient starts selling sex for money (drugs) at the age of 12, she starts drinking when she is 11 and smoking hash when she is 12 and then takes everything she can get her hands on. She sells sex for money from the age of 12-16 and then uses sex as self-harm.

Journal entry woman SAIS 4
The patient says that she is addicted to always being in a relationship because of her low self-esteem. She has been sexually active since she was 16 and she often has sex with men she does not want to have sex with because they show attention or because she feels sorry for them. She seeks out the men online and she becomes overwhelmed by receiving so much attention. She has no control and does not know where to draw the line.

Sublimation

SAIS grade 3-6
In psychoanalysis, people talk about sublimating their traumas, transforming their forbidden drive impulses into something creative. Sublimation is actually a defense but also works therapeutically. Brunet (2007) is an artist and survivor of ritual abuse of incest. In her thesis, she highlights how trauma and art are portrayed. The artist can get lost in their inner world, as an important part of the healing process. Brunet describes creation as a healing process; when the work is finished, the memories are uncovered and incorporated, which in turn can lead to the artist's drive to produce new works of art being reduced. She describes the possibility that some artists in such cases choose not to face the psychological content of their own work so as not to lose the impulse to create. Creating and painting can be a powerful exercise for victims of incest and survivors of sexual abuse and should be done with caution. Perpetrators, known and unknown, unconscious memories and fears can emerge, which the patient is sometimes not ready for. As a therapist, I was present on one occasion when a group member with experience of incest was paralyzed with fear when he painted his childhood traumas and the unconscious became conscious. We had to tear up and stamp on the drawing so that he would get out of his feeling of powerlessness and the experience of being persecuted. What appeared in the painting became a perse-

cuting object. Brunet describes that the artist is always narcissistic to some extent, the work is about themselves, their history and experiences. Sometimes it can take years before she understands her own artwork and can then feel shame that her innermost feelings have been exposed to the outside world. This is reminiscent of the feelings that are aroused when my patients look at pictures they painted as children, they can feel great sadness that no one saw what they painted, when they lacked the words to tell. When art is used as a therapeutic method, one often sees different shapes or lines, colors that are exaggerated to their proportional size or appearance. Newton; referenced in Brunet, (2007) believes that the artist goes through his trauma in an almost oceanic feeling and where all events come to the right place and the fragmentation is thus dissolved. Which in turn eliminates the feeling of guilt and anxiety. Brunet further argues that by having one's own agency when creating shapes and proportions, a sense of control is found in contrast to the loss of control that one experienced when the original event occurred. Which leads to one being able to remember one's trauma from a concentrated aesthetic purpose, the question becomes how can I reproduce my trauma aesthetically instead of trying to remember every moment. Bodily memories, or the condition of how the body remembers what the mind has forgotten, becomes central to the process.

Journal entry woman SAIS 6 DID
The patient sends her art to

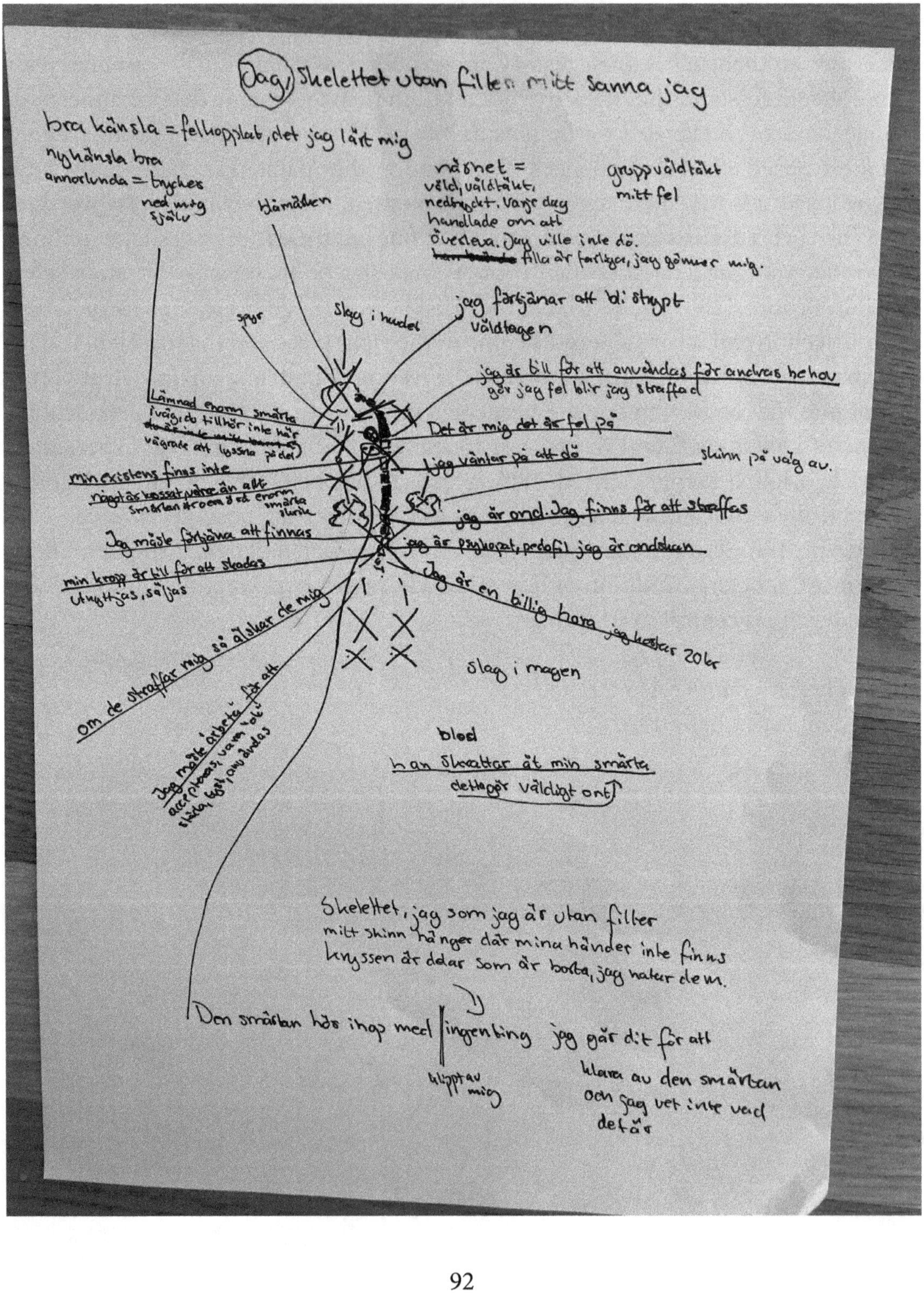
Jag Skelettet utan filter mitt sanna jag
bra känsla = felkopplat, det jag lärt mig
grupp våldtäkt
mitt fel
Jag ville inte dö.
spyr
slag i huvudet
jag förtjänar att bli
jag är till för att användas för andras behov
gör jag fel blir jag straffad
Lämnad enorm smärta
Det är mig det är fel på
Jag väntar på att dö
skinn på väg av.
min existens finns inte
jag är ond. Jag finns för att straffas
Jag måste förtjäna att finnas
jag är psykopat, pedofil jag är ondskan
min kropp är till för att skadas
utnyttjas, säljas
Jag är en billig hora
om de straffar mig så älskar de mig
slag i magen
blod
han skrattar åt min smärta
det gör väldigt ont
Skelettet, jag som jag är utan filter
mitt skinn hänger där mina händer inte finns
Den smärtan hör ihop med ingenting
jag går dit för att
klara av den smärtan
och jag vet inte vad
det är
klipp av
mig

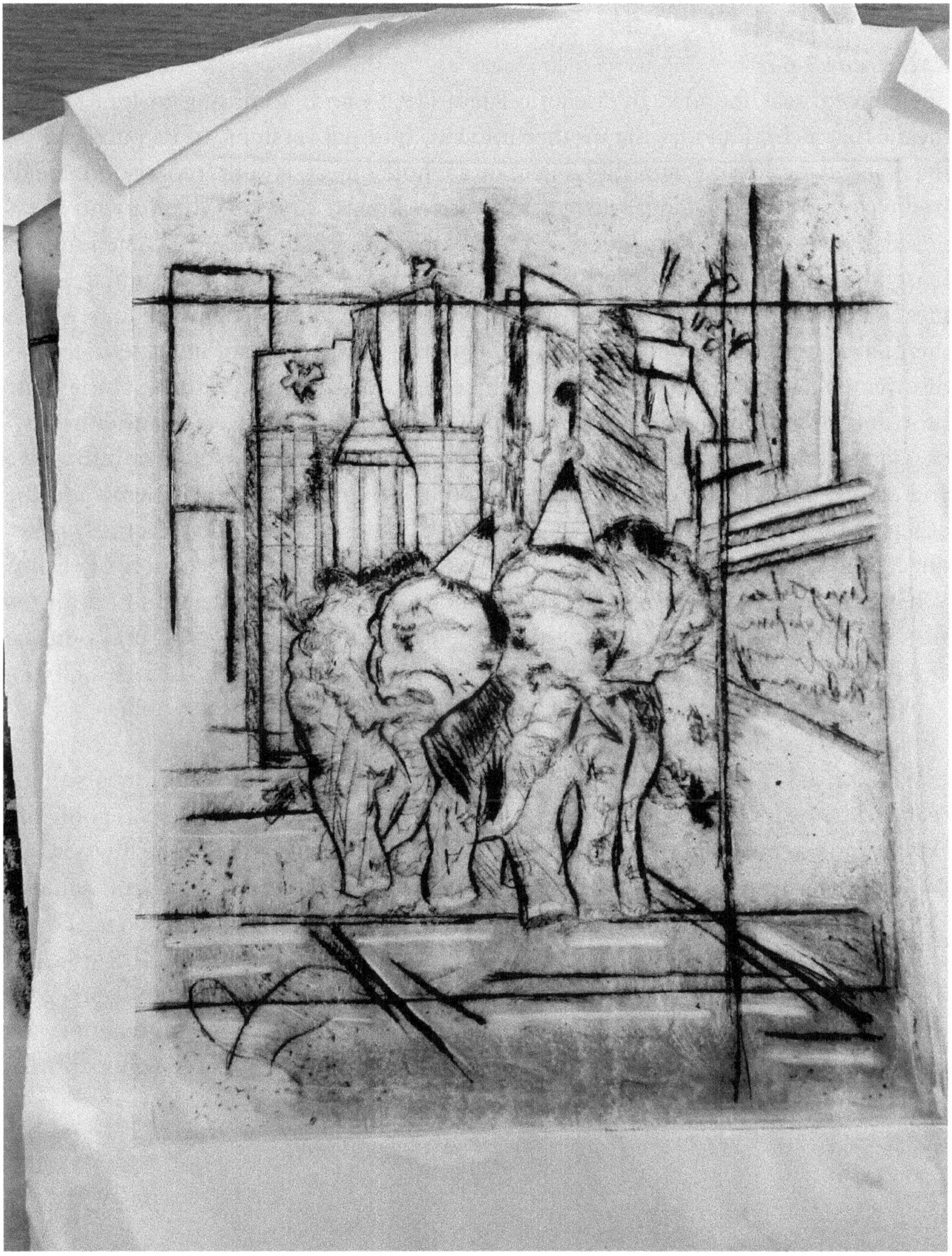

Splitting of the self

SAIS grade 3-6

The concept was founded by Melanie Klein (1929) and, according to Igra (2002), means that a child divides the mother into two internal versions. In its purest form, the object, whether it is a partial object or a whole object, is split into a good, idealized part and an evil, dangerous version (McWilliams, 2011). The child who is exposed divides the world into good and bad with a lack of ambivalence. When the defense is active in an adult, the patient often has a lack of object constancy, which means that there is a difficulty in bringing together contradictory feelings within themselves or others. Adults who exhibit splitting of the self can be experienced as disoriented and contradictory, people can be described as dead and alive at the same time, abrupt changes in the way they speak. Often the parents have become either evil or good or one of them is idealized or devalued. In society we are divided into an we and a they, it can be tempting to designate one group as a clear evil enemy and the others as the righteous who fight against it. The defense often works effectively to reduce anxiety and maintain self-esteem, but always involves a distortion of reality. When the perpetrator is the child's guardian, the child is dependent on him for his survival. Then the child can divide the father into the evil father who preys on the child and the kind father who helps the child with his homework (Donalek, 2001). Separate worlds arise, a nightworld *and* one dayworld *life*. Separate bodies, a head world and a headless world. The body becomes mute and dead, buried alive, rejected, excluded from the inside out. For many incest survivors, it is an enormous pain to realize that the mother probably suspected or could have stopped what was going on. But to come to that realization, they need to stop their idealization of the mother and can no longer split their reality. Only then can we begin to examine what it actually looked like and what the mother's possible motives for her denial consisted of (Freyd, 1996). In the case of negative transference in trauma treatments, the patient will split and assign the therapist different roles such as the perpetrator, the bystander, the victim or the rescuer. As a psychotherapist, a strong, loving hold is required here as the transference will come and go throughout the entire treatment (Wolterstorff & Grassmann, 2013).

Dissociation

SAIS grades 1-6

I will largely devote the rest of the book to explaining and delving into various dissociative states, experiences, and DID as a diagnosis. Dissociation is often interpreted as a defense mechanism, when a patient unconsciously tries to protect themselves from being overwhelmed by a traumatic situation. The patient needs to temporarily protect themselves by avoiding the present because they cannot handle a traumatic situation consciously. When the patient learns to dissociate in traumatic situations, the individual can often arbitrarily respond to other situations by escaping from them via dissociation Gentile, et al., (2013); referenced in Cortez, (2022). Dissociation is a way of separating oneself from reality and can create unpleasant feelings as one can feel cut off, have increased concentration or become activated or daydream. Dissociation is a defense that we all use sometimes in a milder form. An escape from reality can be via alcohol or drugs. In everyday life, this can happen when we relax and disappear for a short while with a glass of wine in our hand after a workweek. Or when we drive to work but forget that we didn't drop off our child at preschool. When we forget something, we can feel dizzy, confused for a short moment, and often it arouses feelings of shame. We often turn the experience into meaningful stories. Dissociation only becomes problematic if you hold on to it for too long and exclude other ways of dealing with reality. Many survivors of childhood sexual abuse can describe hours, sometimes days, disappearing when they are in a state of dissociation. They feel numb and have fragmentary memories of the lost time. They have functioned in a way, gone to the doctor, taken the bus and bought food, but feel that it happened without their control. In dissociation, you lose complete integration of your consciousness, your identity, your memories and experience a lack of perception. Discontinuity and dissociation from one's own thoughts, memories, surroundings, activities and identity are signs of dissociative symptoms. Dissociation allows the patient to escape their day uncontrollably, which usually makes it difficult for them in everyday life. Simply put, dissociation is nature's last resort, the body's own protection against threatening and overwhelming situations. If incest survivors and victims of sexual violence had not had access to dissociation, they would probably not have survived their childhood. Dissociative states can be described as a third reality, an inner world that is visualized, listened to with its own emotional life and perceived as real (Kluft, 1998, 2000; referenced in Howell 2011).

Journal entry woman SAIS 5
The patient says that she can cognitively disappear for long periods of time, not remember meetings with others and shut down.

Journal entry woman SAIS 5 DID
She describes the dissociation as her blinking and then there is a new image.

Division

Dissociation is a way of dividing an event and oneself, in order to survive. When something is linked, it is associated, dissociation (diss association) is its opposite, something is separate. According to Boon (2017), there are two types of dissociative personalities or dissociative states. The first state is that parts function in everyday life and the second is that parts remain in the trauma period, holding traumatic memories, emotions and bodily sensations. For an inexperienced therapist, it can be difficult to distinguish dissociative parts and ego-states (division of experiences and experiences into different ego states) parts. All dissociative parts are ego-state parts but not all ego-state parts are dissociative parts. The difference is that ego-state parts maintain a sense of belonging to the person as a whole. In ego-state division, the patient knows that the different parts exist and they know each other, unlike in DID when the patient may be unaware of having different parts. Dissociative parts have their own sense of identity, self-representations, which means a sense of self, autobiographical memories and their own personal experiences. Dissociative parts also have a sense of I, me and mine, a first-person perspective. Different dissociative parts experience different events in different ways. Dissociation can be explained as a neurobiological and mental defense that is activated to survive what would otherwise not be possible to survive. It can be described as a way for the brain and soul to divide an event or itself, to protect itself from the total fear or horror of the experience. Janet, quoted in Healey (1993), described dissociation as the separation of psychological functions that are usually related. A patient describes herself as a broken mirror that has been shattered into several parts.

Dissociation in the body

In dissociation, a person may sleepwalk, be absent-minded, have forgetfulness, depersonalization (the feeling of looking at one's own body from a distance), derealization or feelings of unreality (as if reality appears like a TV show or inside a snow globe), be immune to the pain of an injury when one's thoughts/mind are elsewhere, the feeling of already *seen*, not recognizing oneself in the mirror, one patient described the entire genital area as dissociated, not being able to remember important parts of one's own life, sudden waves of unexplained strong emotions, hypnotic states and dreams. Dissociation can also be experienced as a self-mutation as *if something had fallen off the body* Classen (1993). The body also has the ability to divide the experience. The most common is perhaps that the person feels that they are leaving the body, can describe the event from the outside, or from above. Depersonalization syndrome could be understood as a condition where one has done so and then has not managed to reintegrate "themselves" with the body. One can also divide or separate different body parts from each other (somatoform dissociative syndrome) or divide and separate the original ability to think and feel simultaneously. Dissociation appears when the child finds himself in unbearable conditions and it is used to shield reality from intolerable pain, fear, horror or a belief that one is about to die. Trost and Levin (1999) describe dissociation as the child's strategies for coping with abuse and the pain it causes by shielding themselves from what is happening. By building a wall between the soul and the body, the child can distance themselves while the abuse is taking place.

In order for a trauma memory to be integrated, the patient needs to know what they have experienced. There are many different trauma methods used to uncover dissociated material. Trauma memories need to be treated clinically, brought up to a certain intensity in the therapy room for the memory to be integrated so as not to trigger flashbacks or triggers in the future. Many times, the patient feels no contact with their body as an adult. It can feel foreign and that parts of the body do not belong to them. They have divided the body, soul and emotional life. The perpetrator could use the body but not the soul. As a psychotherapist in sexual trauma, I have heard countless stories about how the patient saw themselves from the outside or from above, stood by and watched when the abuse occurred. For the small child, it is vital to be able to be outside their body instead of inside it during a particular traumatic experience. Adults who were exposed to sexual abuse in childhood can develop dissociation as a habitual reaction to everyday stresses. Even minor events such as a loud noise, an unpleasant smell, someone raising their voice, or a light touch can put the patient in a dissociative state. Biological research on brain activity during provocation of traumatic memories shows that intense emotions experienced when the memory is encoded are not encoded in such a way that they can be retold according to a narrative structure. Instead, the memories are disjointed islands or states that include bodily somatic reactions, feelings, and images. The memories become countless *events.*The prominent feature of bodily memories is that they occur frequently, both in the past and in the present, and that their power does not fade over time. Intrusive memories, which are usually referred to as flashbacks, involve intense traumatic memories that are not bound in time and that continue to influence experiences in the present (Van der Kolk, 2014).

If you do not remember certain parts of what happened during your childhood due to dissociation, what evidence can you find in such cases to find out about it? According to Miller, (2014) there is evidence through flashbacks because this is when the patient relives parts of their abuse that are in the unconscious. There may also be evidence in body memories. For example, many patients can relive body memories of being raped as a child or being burned with cigarettes. However, it is more difficult to trust body memories than narrative memories, as they often emerge involuntarily.

Journal entry woman SAIS 5 DID
She says her body is suspended from the waist to the knees.

Journal entry woman SAIS 4
During trauma treatment, the patient describes how the groin tenses, it freezes and rushes, the lower abdomen tenses, the sadness sits in the heart and throat.

Amnesia

Memory and our ability to narrate in detail develops throughout life. At about three years of age, children can give short, accurate descriptions of self-experienced events that are close in time. At about five years of age, they can give descriptions of when, where and how something happened and who was involved. The longer time goes by, the more difficult it is to remember details. Traumatic memories, however, are stored in a different way, which means that children can often describe traumatic events both correctly and in detail. If you are exposed to the same type of abuse, by the same person in the same environment on repeated occasions, you tend to remember fewer details; children, just like adults, remember how things used to be (Barnafrid National Knowledge Centre). According to Dahlström-Lannes, (1994); Kwarnmark & Tidefors, (1999); Svedin and Banck, (2002), after the abuse, the child can pretend as if they were dreaming or sleeping when it happened, or that the perpetrator was another person. The strategy is for survival but must not be confused with fantasies about real crimes. Vulnerable children often live in a pseudo-world and are forced to live a lie. Dissociation involves a kind of parallel ownership but at the same time a non-ownership of the experience, part of you owns the experience but part does not. Memories can be experienced as non-integrated, feelings and behaviors as alien, that they do not belong to you (Boon, Steele & Van der Hart, 2012). Dissociative symptoms can be characterized by disturbances or that you experience your consciousness as incoherent, problems with memory, your identity, feelings, perception, body image or problems with behavior. Dissociative symptoms can be ranked from mildly separated from your surroundings to severely separated from your surroundings with identity fragmentation. Dissociation is a way for the body to defend itself when the fight/flight response is impossible (Schröder, Nick, Richter-Appelt and Briken, 2018). More unusual states include near-death experiences and feeling one with the universe. Dissociative amnesia from traumatic events is more common when the caregivers are those involved in the abuse and if it has had to remain a secret Freyd, (1996); referenced in Miller, (2014). Research suggests that each sub-personality has a cluster of autobiographical memories and when one part is active, memories associated with that part become available and memories belonging to other parts become unavailable. Which explains amnesia.

A child who has experienced sexual abuse in a surreal, dream-like state may begin to question their own memories. Whose reality is really true, the child's own or the adult's? (Hedlund, 1996). The feeling of unreality is further reinforced if the child has been under the influence of substances, such as sleeping pills, during the abuse. They may ask themselves, "Did this really happen?" and insist that it is not true. An event can be divided or separated partially or completely from the conscious self (partial or complete dissociative amnesia). When this happens, parts of an event, or the entire sequence of events, are not remembered. It is also common for the person to describe only seeing fragments of the event, such as parts of still images or fragments. There is also evidence in dreams, which can represent our previous experiences, among other things. In mind control, the perpetrators know that dreams contain clues to our past, so they can tell children when they ask about memories that it was just a dream. There are also clues in art such as sublimation, especially in spontaneous works of art, the victim can find indications of trauma that manifests itself in art. But the best indicator of past trauma according to Miller is dissociated material. When different parts or identities take over executively (executive and active), other parts are unaware. If one part takes over without the host part being aware of that part, it is called one-way amnesia. Within a DID system, internal identities or parts may become prone to suddenly take over executive control of the system, which leads to it rejecting the part that was previously in control. This generally results in amnesia in the part that was previously in control, which has been rejected during the time that the new part has taken control. This is called full dissociation Dell, (2009); referenced in Howell, (2011).

Journal entry woman SAIS 4
The woman has dissociative memories of who her abuser is. He has been hiding in the shadows for so long now.

Journal entry woman SAIS 6
The patient is drugged and sees a man stroking the girl's (about 2.5 years old) hair after a prolonged assault by four perpetrators. Now you will soon be able to sleep. This is really just a dream.

A first fragmentation

Many times the patient may experience that their memories have happened to someone else, this may be because it has happened to another part of the patient. A typical example when explaining parts and fragmentation in a trauma is that it is a little girl who sees the abuse from the roof and looks at another little girl who is raped by her father (Ross, 1989; referenced in Howell, 2011). Then there are two little girls who have different consciousnesses. The first little girl can go to school the next day without knowing that she was raped by her father the night before. Those memories are within the girl who saw herself from the roof. In the book Miss America by Day (2003), Marilyn Van Derbur, who was Miss America in 1958, describes that she was both a day girl and a night girl. The day girl did not know about the night girl until she got older and started psychotherapy. According to Miller (2014), several studies show that dissociated memories that are forgotten and then recovered are just as likely to be true as those that have always been remembered.

In traumatic dissociation, the parts are separated by strong barriers so that one part is not aware of the abuse or feelings that another part experiences. The part that goes to school is not aware of the abuse that happens at home in the family, those memories are kept in another part of the child. As a protection or defense, in order to continue developing. Sometimes the child cannot even remember the abuse that happened the night before. Which explains why children cannot describe the crimes they were subjected to afterwards during, for example, a police investigation.

A Supreme Court ruling states that the child's story needs to be clear, long, vivid, logical, rich in detail, proven to be truthful in important details, and free from inaccuracies, contradictions, exaggerations, difficult-to-explain moments, lack of consistency, poor coherence, or hesitation in crucial parts (GP, 2025). What the court requires is completely opposite to how dissociative memories are encoded, stored, and retold.

Many children are phobically afraid of entering the part that is being abused when they are in another part that is not being abused. A patient (9 years old) who had been sexually abused by an outsider screamed loudly or sat completely mute and isolated in herself when the parents, together with the therapist, tried to approach the material. Dissociative splitting is an adaptive ability that allows the child to continue living his life, despite ongoing trauma (Miller, 2014).

Journal entry woman SAIS 4

The patient in trauma therapy goes back to the memory as a scene where she sees herself from the outside, from a corner of the room. The child she sees goes up to the man's waist, she changes perspective in the therapy room and becomes the child in the memory. She holds her face in the therapy room as she becomes the child in the memory and it hurts her head as the man holds her head tightly during an oral rape.

Journal entry woman SAIS 4

The patient has been in support sessions for a year before she is referred to trauma treatment where the patient is not given access to her memories. She has fragments of several assaults such as the smell of hay, wet leaves, seeing her pants pulled down, hearing the sound of a fly being pulled down behind her. Everything before and after the fragments is black and the material is dissociated. The moment of surprise in the rapes that her perpetrator used made her immediately go from fear to horror and end up in freeze. In the treatment we go from the fragments of wet leaves to a dissociated part that sees the assault from above. The part sees a man's body lying in the forest above a small child. The part can then play back in the memory and we see how the assault begins. At the next session the patient has regained the memory of how she feels after the assault was over. How the perpetrator says that it wasn't that bad and that's what you do if you love each other. He was 40 years older than her. She was 7 years old.

What affects the degree of dissociation?

Christine Courtois (1996) writes in her book *Healing the Incest wound* about various factors within sexual abuse that influence and reinforce the degree of dissociation. The severity of the patient's symptoms is associated with a number of factors regarding how the abuse picture has looked.

How long you have been exposed

Trickett, Reiffman, Horowitz & Putnam (1997) report that the outcome of the trauma becomes worse the longer the abuse has been going on and the more frequent it has been. The age at which the abuse started and how long it continued is important for the patient's degree of traumatization. According to (Kaplow & Widom, (2007); Maniglio, (2009); McCellen et al., (1996); referenced in Ventus, Antfolk & Salo, (2016), the risk of psychopathology is higher the earlier the sexual abuse begins in the child's life. According to Homburger-Erikson (1971), the child's development is divided into five phases in which the child has different needs and ways of expressing themselves. In the first phase between birth and 1.5 years, trust in oneself and the world is built up, the prerequisite for this is good relationships with secure individuals, primarily parents are needed to create a basic trust. Bowlby (2010) believes that the attachment to parents is strongest during the first year of life but takes place throughout childhood. In the second phase between 1.5–3 years, children's curiosity is aroused and they demonstrate their self-worth by wanting to do things on their own. When the child is exposed to danger or uncertainty, they return to the attachment figure, the secure base for comfort and protection, which leads to the child being able to handle powerful emotions (Bowlby, 2010). In the third phase, 3–6 years, the child's motor skills, memory and ability to identify things develop. Language also develops, which increases the child's understanding of concepts. Self-confidence and trust in others create initiative-taking children who dare to explore their environment to a greater extent. In phase four, 6–12 years, the interest in learning new things and being proactive together with others in the environment such as parents, playmates or school staff develops. Self-esteem and pride increase through encouragement for the child. In the fifth phase, between 12–20 years, the child goes from teenager to adult. Here, the teenager must free themselves symbolically by gathering all their anger, aggression and power to be able to leave their parents. The child must always believe that the place they are going to is better than the one they are leaving. Which means that they need to devalue their parents to a certain extent and idealize themselves. Through contact and interaction with others a secure identity is formed. If the teenager has not been confirmed, it can result in uncertainty about the personality and the development of a destructive view of identity (Holmburger-Eriksson, 1971).

In the case of single abuses, treatment only needs to take into account the child's cognitive functioning level at the specific time/times. Abuses such as incest often continue over a longer period and thus involve a higher frequency of abuse and longer exposure over time. Shelvin, Dorahy, & Adamson (2007) believe that general population studies have shown that there is a correlation between early traumas and the development of psychotic experiences and psychotic symptoms. Infants are particularly susceptible to automation of experiences because the brain is plastic and prone to change. The experiences that the child is involved in dictate how associations in the brain are built. As a result of the neural structures of the brain and the associations between them, conscious memories are undeveloped during the first year of life. There is practically no possibility for the individual to later recapitulate how these early experiences were acquired. Here, memory researchers distinguish between *implicit and explicit*, unconscious and conscious memories Field, (2000); referenced in Broberg, Granqvist, Ivarsson & Risholm Mothander, (2015). In the case of early abuse, the patient often does not remember any life before the abuse, but they have always been part of their world of experience. This usually means attachment trauma as the abuse was most likely carried out by someone close to the child, such as a close relative or caregiver. According to Svedin and Blanck (2002), the most common symptoms for children who have been exposed between the ages of 0 and 6 are PTSD, anxiety, nightmares and inappropriate sexual behavior. Since the early abuse is not quantifiable for the patient, physical bodily sensations are created and the body becomes the one keeping score and the world of experience implies that people are dangerous. At school age, many bodily changes occur naturally and the transition from a child's body to a teenager often arouses feelings of shame, which are reinforced in the case of sexual abuse. According to Svedin and Blanck (2002), the most common symptoms for sexually abused children aged 7–12 are nightmares, fear, aggression, mental illness, problems at school and hyperactivity. Several of my patients describe that their prepubertal development was followed with great interest by the abusive parent, ridiculed or became the object of the perpetrator's targeted attraction. It can also arouse shame with early menstruation. In adolescence, sexuality develops side by side with the abuse and many describe feelings of shame in relation to voluntary sex. According to Svedin and Blanck (2002), the symptoms for abused children aged 13–18 are self-harm, substance abuse, depression, suicidal tendencies, illegal acts and promiscuity. According to Erika Johansson Laukka, senior lecturer in ageing, the sense of time is elastic and is experienced more stretchable when we are young. The moment lasts longer according to the proportional theory of Paul Janet, (1897); referenced in DN, which means that three weeks for a five-year-old feels like a year for a 54-year-old. The older you get, the smaller part of life a year makes up proportionally, which makes it feel as if time passes faster. Many of my patients testify that as small children they felt that the abuse lasted forever, they felt endless and as if it never ended. One patient said that it felt as if I was lying there for 1000 years.

How frequent the abuse has been

How frequent the abuse was, the degree of contact, the use of force, the age of the victim when it began and the closeness of the relationship to the perpetrator affect how negative the effects of childhood sexual abuse are generated Beitchman et al., (1991); Roosa et al., (1999); Tyler, (2002); referenced in Ventus, Antfolk & Salo, (2016). In a meta-analysis of 62 studies where 220 different effects of sexual abuse were observed in 14,494 cases. The researchers found a correlation that sexual abuse within the family had a higher probability of starting early in the child's life and occurred more frequently than abuse by an outside perpetrator. The earlier the abuse started, the more experience of other variables such as longer duration, more coercion and psychological distress. One possible explanation that the researchers address is that young children are not as easy to access if it is not one's own or in the immediate family. The results also showed that the earlier the first episode of abuse was, the higher the quantity of abuse. Children who have experienced a higher quantity of sexual abuse in childhood also have a higher risk of suffering more ACE's adverse childhood experiences. Lena Morin, who has written the book Never could he kill me, is herself an incest survivor, who founded nxtME. She pointed out during #metoo that it is positive that we pay attention to sexual violence but noted the danger of equating milder sexual abuse with incest. There is a significant difference between being the victim of one rape as an adult and a hundred rapes as a child.

Penetrating assault

According to Tyler (2002), more intrusive, penetrating abuse leads to more negative effects for the victim than less intrusive abuse. The association between the degree of coercion and the degree of contact means that penetrative abuse requires coercion to gain sufficient control over the victim (Burton, 2000). In purely instrumental terms, more violence is required in penetrating assaults to be able to carry out the act. Male perpetrators where the perpetrator is a biological father or stepfather use penetration more often and the survivors suffer more long-term and serious consequences as the abuse usually begins at an early age (Rathsman, 2001).

Journal entry woman SAIS 5 DID
She accesses the memory of penetration and a pressure on her back, as if she is about to be crushed.

Journal entry woman SAIS 4
She feels terrified about coming into contact with the memory, it hurts like period pain, inside around the ovaries. He wants her to relax, guides her through, she is very tense, it hurts when he inserts a dildo. The patient feels that he enjoys the power, he likes that she is tense and afraid. He speaks soothingly to her.

Degree of violence, coercion and intimidation

Roland Summit (1983) explains the phenomenon of children's silence in the face of ongoing sexual abuse with child *sexual abuse accommodation syndrome,* the average child never asks and never tells. He describes a model of how a child learns to accept their situation and how they can survive ongoing sexual abuse. The child knows that there is no way out and nowhere to run. Non-exposed children develop normal emotional resilience, which means a long-term ability for the child to handle changes and continue to develop. However, exposed children instead learn to conform to their reality, which includes sexual abuse. According to Hedlund (1996), the child can reinterpret the understanding of the abuse into something everyday, such as that all fathers do this to their children. This reinterpretation occurs due to the ability to split, the child pushes away and forgets her own feelings. The child's perception of the ongoing sexual abuse changes over time. A ten-year-old girl does not have the same perception of sexual abuse as when she was three. The child puts the experiences of the sexual abuse in relation to the effects if they were to reveal what is really happening. According to Summit (1983), the child goes through five stages: a) secrets, b) helplessness, c) feeling trapped and compliant, d) the child waits to tell, e) the child withdraws.

Those who practice sexual violence use various strategies to silence a child before the abuse, such as isolating the victim, submissive behavior or lies. During the abuse, the perpetrator uses physical violence, threats or humiliation. Then, after the abuse, the perpetrator denies or hides and minimizes the victim's injuries. The perpetrator blames the victim or refuses to take responsibility for the violence by suppressing or breaking down the victim's resistance (Wade, 2010). It is very difficult for the child to reveal what has happened, there is one or more perpetrators who invade the body and besiege it. Carlsson (2004) describes it as a warlord who has declared ownership and then continues to live his life inside the child. The child does not understand what is happening but still knows that life is in danger when he whispers, "We're just going to have a little fun" or "Only I can love you." The child knows that this cannot be talked about. It is a law, a law of secrecy followed by gifts that create a debt of gratitude followed by persuasion and threats.

Threats of exclusion are society's ultimate form of sanction used to reinforce the individual's adaptation and thereby ensure cultural homogeneity. Being excluded and being different arouses feelings of shame and leads the individual to adapt to prevailing norms. In the case of incest, the perpetrator is a person the child knows, has a relationship with, and is often in a hierarchically inferior position to. The child's dependence is greater the younger she is; if she were to tell, she risks being excluded from important life-determining relationships Jaggar, (2000); referenced in Carlsson, (2004). For children who have been exposed to pedophilic circles, there are additional factors that can contribute to a higher level of emotional and social trauma. These factors consist of serious threats, documentation via photo and video, and the number of perpetrators; the greater the number of perpetrators, the greater the impact on the child's trust in adults (Svedin and Banck, 2002).

Journal entry woman SAIS 4
The patient says that her perpetrator has said that he has raped and killed several women in the past. He says that the woman's vagina becomes completely warm just before she dies, he strangles her while raping her to relive his previous experiences.

Journal entry woman SAIS 6 DID
The man is still angry and calls her a whore, a slut and other insulting words. He then pulls her down to the floor and puts his foot on her chest, she is lying on the floor on her back. He says he can push and crush her chest if he wants and she will die. He asks her if she is scared.

Journal entry woman SAIS 5 DID
She has child parts that act as voices that say she can't tell because she's not safe and the perpetrator can still hurt her. I say that the perpetrator can't hurt her today and that part remains in the trauma period, the abuse happened 30 years ago.

Journal entry woman SAIS 4
Her father often bought her gifts after the abuse, from Barbies when she was younger to makeup when she was older. He trained her to be quiet by playing various games with insignificant objects.

A male perpetrator

The perpetrator is usually someone close to the child. The perpetrator can be a close or distant friend of the family, but most often fathers or other father figures (National Association of Support Centers Against Incest, 2023). Research shows that sexual abuse with the biological father as the perpetrator is associated with a younger age when the abuse starts, a longer duration and more abuse situations compared to other sexual abuses Kendall-Tackett et al., (1993); Tricket, Noll & Putnam, (2011). Petterson's (2013) study on the experience of shame after incest showed that male perpetrators in the form of a guardian were more associated with feelings of guilt, as the victim considered themselves complicit in the abuse. Shame was reserved for the mothers. Respondents in the study experienced more shame towards their mothers than their fathers. They were preoccupied with the thought of why their mother had not protected them or that they had let their mother down. According to Dahlström-Lannes (1994), boys have a harder time than girls admitting the feelings of powerlessness and helplessness that sexual abuse generates and can therefore, if they are victimized by a man, identify with the perpetrator. When men abuse boys, there is a tendency to keep this a secret because they believe that they themselves have become or will be regarded as homosexual if the perpetrator is a man. According to Gill & Tutty, (1997); referenced in Tidefors Andersson (2002), the conflict for boys is reinforced by seeing themselves as victims in relation to society's expectations of masculinity. The more traditional a society is regarding gender roles, the greater the tendency for boys not to talk about sexual abuse. The number of male perpetrators also has a major impact on the development of dissociation.

The closeness of the relationship

Fergusson & Mullen, (1999); referenced in Svedin and Banck, (2002) point out that usually the perpetrator is known to the child and is in the child's immediate environment. Biological paternal incest is the most common and the one with the most serious consequences (Gomes et al. 2014). According to Ullman, Filipas, Townsend, Starzynski, (2007); referenced in Schröder, Nick, Richter-Appelt and Briken, (2018), recent studies have shown that children who have been sexually abused within the family had more severe PTSD symptoms. The father is intended to be protective, caring, encouraging, supportive and nurturing of the child but instead becomes the one who exploits and exposes the child to abuse Fischer & McDonald, (1998); Wolfe, (2006); referenced in Baker (2015). Criminologist Kutchinsky, (1994); referenced in Tidefors Andersson, (2002) claims that most abuse by an unknown person is reported, but the closer the relationship, the fewer people report. According to Sheinberg & Fraenkel, (2001); referenced in Kluft, (2010) the closeness of the relationship between the victim and the perpetrator complicates the trauma. Relational trauma leads to a significant loss of trust in other people and increases anger, pain and confusion in family relationships. This changes the child's trust in close relationships in general and the child's integral negative internalized beliefs about oneself in relation to others. In many cases when the incest is revealed, the victim is excluded from the family and distrusted, the family sides with the perpetrator to protect themselves, which becomes a retraumatization for the victim. Several studies show that the consequences of sibling incest are as great as when it is an adult perpetrator Cyr et al., (2002); McVeigh, (2003); referenced in Benisimon & Mashiach, (2021). Although sibling incest is considered one of the most common forms of sexual abuse of children, the phenomenon has received little attention in research Phillips-Green, (2002); Smith & Israel, (1987). Few studies have focused on the significance that distinguishes normal sexual play between children/siblings from sibling incest. When play turns into abuse with dimensions that include age difference between the children, type of sexual behavior (touching each other to penetration), what motivates the behavior (exploratory to wanting to cause harm) or whether there has been reciprocity in the relationship Caffaro & Conn-Caffaro, (1998); DeJong, (1989); Finkelhor, (1980); Weihe & Herring, (1991); referenced in Katz & Hamama, (2015). There are major contradictions in the research regarding age differences in Cyr et al., (2002); referenced in Katz & Hamama, (2015) study from (2002) shows that the median age difference is 5.3 years between the victim and the perpetrator. Other studies have shown situations where the perpetrator may be younger than the victim. The age difference between siblings in incest may be less relevant because in traditional contexts in patriarchal family structures, it is men who possess more power Caffaro & Conn-Carraro, (1998); Laviola, (1992); Pierce & Pierce, (1990); referenced in Katz & Hamama, (2015). Regarding what motivates the behavior of the perpetrator who abuses his sibling, studies show that there are psychiatric diagnoses, a variety of problematic behaviors, previous experience of sexual or psychological abuse, exposure to pornography, exposure to domestic violence, more aggressive family dysfunctions and a sexualized home environment Latzman, Vijoen, Scalora & Ullman, (2011); referenced in Katz & Hamama, (2015). But most commonly, it is when an older child entering adolescence abuses a younger sibling. When the perpetrator is a family member and the rest of the family either ignores or encourages the abuse, the child will lose their faith in the world as a safe place and their perception of being protected from evil Lev-Wiesel, (2015); referenced in Benismon & Mashiach, (2021).

Passive or willing participation

According to Lingåker (2017), sexual abuse of children is characterized by an adult or someone older than the child exploiting the child's dependent position to satisfy their own sexual needs. The child is made the object of actions that she/he is not mature enough for or can give informed consent to. Ernst et al., (1985) believe that even if the sexual relationship with a child occurs in a soft, manipulative and seemingly loving manner, this does not mean that the child is not harmed. Sexual relationships between children and adults are always, at all times, an abuse, regardless of whether the child has apparently participated or taken the sexual initiative. It is always the adult's responsibility to draw boundaries. The child's adaptation to the abuse situation counteracts the possibility of seeing through its function, namely to satisfy a need of the perpetrator. Even if girls and boys perceive the abuse differently in terms of content, they have the same tendencies to adapt to it (Hedlund, 1996). During long periods of ongoing incest, the child will develop coping mechanisms to cope with the anxiety that arises in the waiting period between assaults. In Finkelhor & Araji's study from (1986) described in A Confused Dynamic, the phase when the assault is over is a calmer time for the perpetrator when the sexual tension, aversion, anxiety and displeasure that he felt before have been reduced. For the child, it is just an uncertain wait for the next opportunity. In order to experience some form of control, the child may initiate an assault himself in anticipation of the next assault in order to at least be able to control when in time it occurs. Several of my patients testify to the fear of going to bed, night terrors in anticipation of being woken up. Children often go to bed before the perpetrator and are often in deep sleep when they wake up during ongoing assaults. Which made them feel confused and experienced feelings of unreality, were they in a nightmare or in reality. To escape the terrifying feeling of waking up during ongoing abuse, they could initiate and approach the perpetrator themselves, which in retrospect arouses feelings of both confusion and shame. Did I want it to happen or was I part of it? The child may also have approached the parent to seek comfort, which has turned into abuse, which in post-constructions can be experienced as if one had sought out the perpetrator. Female perpetrators often weave the abuse into otherwise nice moments such as storytime or games, sadistic clinging tickling games that go overboard and end in sexual abuse. Or moments of care such as showering the child who is caressed, gets an erection and where the desire is projected onto the child. A hug in a family where incest occurs is never just a hug. The confused dynamics of natural bodily reactions can be experienced as willing participation. Incest is repetitive, like a learning process, and the adaptation means learning what the perpetrator likes, what moves are included, and how to perform them. Children are trained to satisfy the perpetrator's expressed sexual needs through penetration training, positions, learning the different moves, and how the perpetrator wants them performed.

Involuntary erotic response

Today, an erotic response is called a non-conforming sexual response. Many people experience a physical response during sexual assault and you can have an orgasm during rape. But it is not a sexual response that can be likened to feeling desire, sexual reciprocity or to including some type of consent or that one enjoys it (Nagoski, 2021). An orgasm is a physiological, involuntary, uncontrolled response to sexual, usually mechanical genital simulation. An orgasm must never be misinterpreted as consent to an assault. Biologically, people react relatively similarly to sexual stimulation. The autonomic nervous system is activated and causes increased breathing, pulse, muscle tension and blood pressure. The increased blood flow to our genitals provides an erection in the man and lubrication in the woman. Physical response to a sexual assault is not consent or a receipt of pleasure, our genitals do not speak about what we like. Through psychoeducation, we need to distinguish/clarify in the therapy room how the body reacted during the assault and their unwillingness to participate. Which is a healing knowledge. It is difficult to understand how one can have an orgasm during a rape, which can lead to confusion. Sex education needs to be developed and the knowledge that the body can react the same way during an assault as during consensual sex needs to be clarified. Experiencing lubrication, getting an erection, stiff nipples, having an orgasm does not necessarily mean that you have given consent. Your body may react one way but you want something else.

In extreme sexual abuse, parts are organically created within the patient that can navigate whatever is expected of them during the abuse. Abusers demand that the victim be molded to serve the abuser's function. Many times, the victim has their first erotic response with the abuser, creating a disturbed ego dystonia (thoughts, feelings, or behavior that contradict a person's self-image) association between the abuse and a sexual erotic response. Later in life, consensual sex or masturbation to experience sexual pleasure can involuntarily lead to flashbacks of the abuse. This often leads to victims feeling sinful, perverted, and unloved. However, victims are not responsible for sensations produced in their bodies during abusive situations, inflicted by their abuser. Such responses do not mean that the victim has sought out the abuser, even if they eventually found ways to escape into the experience. Which can sometimes mean that the victim may have experienced sexual sensations during the abuse. An insight that is often followed by feelings of guilt and shame. Many patients later re-enter situations in adult life with consensual sex that are reminiscent of abuse situations in, for example BDSM (collective name for bondage, discipline, dominance, submission and masochism) but then with stop words, consent and self-control. When one remembers situations from childhood abuse and their response in adult life, it is simply a product of associative memories. Memories that are similar to each other and share certain elements and are associated with each other in our memory paths. Victims can, after abuse, in adult life slowly begin to associate sexual pleasure with activities of their own choosing. The trick, according to Lacter (2022), is to use self-care instead of judging oneself through feelings of shame in the moments when our mind is drawn to memories of abuse.

Journal entry woman SAIS 6 DID

Some parts is 6 years old and describe that nothing inside her exists. She doesn't know what feelings are except pain and orgasms. She likes orgasms because then it feels like she's flying or like an explosion in space.

Guilt, shame, disgust

Guilt and shame can often be traced to a subjective experience of having done something wrong, having failed at something (guilt) or of the feeling of being wrong or a failure (shame). When it comes to sexual violence, it is more the rule than the exception that perpetrators say or show in various ways that what is happening is the victim's fault. For a confident adult it can be relatively easy to understand that it is a lie, that it was clearly the perpetrator who did wrong and bears both the guilt and the shame of the crime committed, although almost everyone still needs help to have this confirmed and consolidated. For a child who is forming his worldview, it is not as easy, even well into adulthood in treatment, the child's internalized beliefs that it is the child, and not the perpetrator, who either does or is, wrong.

The variations in how guilt, shame and disgust can interact are endless. A person can feel guilty about feeling shame and disgust, or feel ashamed of their feelings of guilt and disgust, or one of the three can be so strong that only one can be felt at a time. What both guilt, shame and disgust have in common is that they all affect the relationship to one's own self, one's own body and one's own being. One's own physical being cannot be run away from. If the intensity of these experiences becomes too strong, my experience is that alienation from one's own body through dissociation becomes the solution the brain uses, when no other solution exists. My experience is that when one breaks dissociation through treatment, one needs to be prepared for the possibility that strong feelings of guilt, shame and disgust, and the accompanying risk of self-destructive behavioral patterns and suicidality, may emerge. My experience is that it can be of great importance for the therapist to understand whether it is guilt, shame or disgust that is the underlying driving force behind destructive behavioral patterns and suicidality and to identify early on how much of destructive behavioral patterns and suicidality is about pure coping mechanisms.

The Shame Compass describes four different ways used to defend oneself against shame. The patient can become a) Withdrawn, which means that one feels resigned, lacks motivation, becomes passive or depressed when experiencing humiliation, b) Avoidant, which leads to over-adaptation to the world, one may constantly perform, become boastful, assertive, shameless and shake off to limit or deny the shame, c) Attack on the self, which means that we devalue, show self-contempt, have poor self-confidence, self-harm or suicide. Here the patient himself becomes the bearer of shame and thus punishes himself to control the feelings of shame, d) Attack directed at others, which means that others have to bear the shame, guilt and anger, one despises, devalues and offends others because of feelings of own inferiority (Nathanson, 1992). According to Tomkins' (2008) theory of affect, shame is considered one of our basic effects. Shame is an emotion that is created early and is awakened within us when we have shown positive affect or interest towards someone else who reacts with distancing. The interaction and how one reflects oneself between the parent and the child is fundamental to the child's emotional development. In the affect-focused therapy ISTDP (Intensive Short Dynamic Psychotherapy), it is primarily the affects that motivate us to act and not the drives that were assumed in psychoanalysis. Recovery in therapy occurs by re-experiencing the underlying emotions and in turn creating new insights in the patient (Bergsten, 2015). In purely physical terms, research shows that shame activates parts of the hypothalamus that, via the endocrine system, affect the individual's fight-or-flight system and the involuntary muscles (Schore, 1998). Darwin, (1872); referenced by Ramberg in the journal Psychotherapy mean that *Blushing is the most peculiar and the most human of all human expressions.* Kjellqvist defines two different types of shame, red and white shame. Red shame, being embarrassed, flaring up in the face, functions as a warning signal and has to do with violating one's own and others' boundaries. That is, when something is embarrassing for us. Kjellqvist (2006) believes that red shame is bloody and throbbing with life, while white shame is deathly pale and of such devastating strength that it drives away all life. White shame is manifested by a lost vitality, the shoulders are pushed forward and downward, the upper body tends to collapse and the head falls forward and downward. The eyes look downward, a protection against seeing or being seen. Affects pass while the shame persists. In Beck Friis's (2009) book *The naked shame,* a more serious shame appears when we feel that our entire functionality is threatened and we are unable to maintain our integrity in front of others. Which is the case for incest survivors and vulnerable children in organized and ritual abuse. The white shame appears when the boundary crossing has already occurred. It is founded when as a child you are not seen or confirmed in that you exist, the child becomes a function for someone else, you have lost the right to exist for the person you are. The white shame means that there is something fundamentally wrong with me as an individual and it cannot be fixed. My patients often make long explanations of everything that is wrong with them, they accumulate all bad decisions or events as evidence of their worthlessness. An unabashed contempt for how they were as children, disgusting, seductive and they deserve everything that happened to them. The white shame is incorporated and explains that it is because there is something so terribly wrong *with them* who have caused their parents to hurt them and not be able to love them. They are unlovable, used up and got what they deserved. Facing and dealing with white shame is one of the most difficult things there is. To awaken even an ounce of their own care to the defenseless child self that they hate is a patient journey. It is often said that shame is the perpetrator's best friend.

Journal entry woman SAIS 3
The patient says that after her abuse was discovered at the age of 11, her mother took her for a virginity check and her father hit her. She describes a lonely childhood without care, love or safe adults.

Journal entry woman SAIS 3
The patient says that it is out of the question for her to tell what happened to her, as she does not want to create a conflict and the perpetrator still comes to family gatherings. She says that her aunt will not believe her and will accuse her of being at fault for sending out signals. She is the only one who bears the shame.

Journal entry man SAIS 3
The patient feels shame throughout his life, "there is something wrong with me, I have always disappointed people."

Journal entry woman SAIS 4
The patient took a bath in her teens with a bruised back, and her mother came in and told her to tell them not to hit you too hard next time.

The Westermarck effect - feeling of disgust

Disgust can be seen as a biological reaction to threats to health. Moldy and spoiled food is a good example of things that arouse disgust. If we have tasted something really disgusting, we often avoid it for a long time, and do everything we can to avoid eating it again. In the case of sexual violence, it is common for the disgust from the event itself to be stored in one's own body, and the victim may become shunned and want to avoid their own body at all costs. Disgust and shame seem to be closely linked, and the combination of disgust and shame towards oneself can seem almost unbearable to harbor. The disgust and the avoidance it creates in itself reduces the possibility of exposure therapy.

Westermarck (1981) highlights an aspect of disgust, in relation to the incest taboo in *The history of human marrige* where he speaks of incest as both a socially taboo and a psychologically biologically conditioned reaction. The instinct of not wanting to have sex with a close relative. He acknowledged that the greatest cost of incest is the reproductive one due to inbreeding but also addressed the aspect of an innate aversion to incest. There, a critical window was suggested that when family members live together in childhood before the age of 6, they are likely to activate a mechanism of sexual aversion between them. Multiple studies have shown that genetically unrelated children who grow up together from birth are unlikely to develop sexual relationships Shepher, (1971); Spiro, (1958); Talmon, (1964); referenced in Pullman, Babchishin & Seto, (2019). In order to develop a dislike for incestuous and avoid incestuous behavior, one needs to be able to identify kinship. Mothers have the evolutionary advantage of being certain that they share 50% of their child's genes by carrying the child and through birth. Genetic relatedness is not a trait that can be directly observed and the father can rarely know for sure that the relationship is established as his partner may have had children with another partner. According to Andersson, (2006); referenced in Pullman, Babchishin & Seto, (2019) it has been shown that 2% of men in the general population are raising a child with whom they do not share genes in uncertainty. According to Heth, Todrand & Johnston, (1999); referenced in Pullman, Babchishin & Seto, (2019) similarity in scents can be a way to distinguish kinship for both animals and humans. Or phenotypical (a trait that is easily observed) similar physical features. According to Apicella & Marlowe, (2004); Burch & Gallup, (2000); referenced in Pullman, Babchishin & Seto, (2019) fathers tend to favor and provide more resources to children who are similar to them. Parents often experience their child's scent as the child enters adolescence as a strong, sweaty scent that arouses disgust in the parent. We experience the scent more strongly than outsiders, as we have a naturally built-in aversion as they develop sexually. Westermarck

(1981) argued that social norms towards incest are an extension of the individual's *own* aversion to the idea that they would act incestuous. By talking about incest, many people are unable to keep internal images from themselves, they unconsciously imagine that they themselves could expose a child or have been exposed by their parents. Westermarck (1981) addressed the fact that it was not only caused by the disapproval of the environment or a legal prohibition, but also stems from the individual's own feelings. This means that when someone talks about incest, it arouses feelings of disgust in the listener. The feeling of disgust is both projected from the person who tells the story and aroused from within the listener himself when listening to stories about incest. Not towards the person who tells the story but towards the act as such.

For the patient, it is healing when the feeling of disgust is neutralized. We do this partly because the therapist is experienced with similar traumas and by talking about what arouses disgust with neutralizing language. By talking about what disgusts us, we remove the charge and intensity of the feeling. Maria Lundberg (2023), who wrote the book You Should Not Bear the Shame for What Happened, says that in therapy she came to the realization that the abuse does not mean that she is disgusting, but that she can be disgusted by the abuse, but that that is a completely different thing.

Incest survivors often experience their bodies as unclean, disgusting, unreal and that the abuse cannot be washed away. A respondent in Dareflod & Nyberg's study from (2010) described themselves as disgusting, disgusting, disgusting, like a tumor, a large walking penis. Finkelhor and Browne (1997) describe that perpetrators often attribute guilt and derogatory negative characteristics to children such as having been promiscuous and seductive. Dareflod and Nyberg (2010) describe that respondents in their study described their bodies as dirty, disgusting, broken and destroyed both inside and out. They walked around with a lump of disgust inside them that could not be removed, felt disgust over body parts such as the genitals and mouth. They said that the perpetrator's scent remained on their bodies, no matter how much they washed themselves, it did not go away. There was also a tangible fear that the abuse had left visible traces on the outside. One patient explained it as if perpetrators were drawn to her like flies on a sugar cube, they feel that she had been exposed and was therefore vulnerable, an easy victim of new abuse. Strong feelings of hatred and disgust can be directed towards one's own body and the abuse makes them despise themselves. Which can then be further understood by the individual controlling their own body or directing visible physical pain towards the body which manifests itself in various self-harming behaviors.

Betrayal, horror and confusion

The betrayal of the person who chooses to harm by exposing someone to sexual violence is often experienced as great and clear when an adult is exposed. My experience is that for children who are exposed, it is much more difficult to see it that way, even when they have become adults. A common interpretation may be that it is not a betrayal – but a righteous act that the child deserves because of their own mistakes. Another common interpretation is that it is not those who expose the child who are betraying, but that it is the world as such that cannot be trusted. It is also common for the confusion and fear to become so great that cognitive conceptualizations of what has happened cannot be made, or that what is happening is so unpredictable that it is not possible to create understandable models of cause and effect and a constant feeling of danger to life and of never being able to be safe instead develops. The confusion during and after sexual violence can be or develop to be minor or total. The greater the fear, the more difficult it is to bring clarity, the greater the confusion, the greater the fear.

The experience and reaction in fear is influenced by both how strongly life-threatening an event is perceived to be. As mentioned earlier, two main tracks can be chosen – fight/flight, or dissociation, although the truth is most often that it is a mixture of both tracks. My experience is that regardless of which track is chosen, memory function is always affected in some way. Working with a timeline, both to stabilize memory function in the present and to anchor and integrate traumatic memories, is effective and safe.

Journal entry man SAIS 5

He walks hand in hand with his coach, walking from the soccer field towards a forest where they usually train at the outdoor gym, it feels like he's happy, it feels easy, it's an outing for the two of them, he's chosen, and special, he says it's a secret, he asks if he trusts him, he says yes, he was happy, the first time, he's more innocent, he looks up and sees that he's happy too, he built up hope, it will get better, we belong together, that he wanted it to happen, that it's my fault and that my family will think I'm disgusting if I tell, no one will believe me.

He undresses him, he sits and looks at his pants, which are pulled down, he says it's a new game, he touches his legs, he thinks he's lying on his back now, he sees treetops, it's windy outside.

From above, in another part, he sees how the man moves mechanically, with his hand higher up, the man looks happy, down on a hard surface, a stone, he lies down with his legs on the edge, he lies on his back, then it jumps to the previous memory, he lies on him, he stands and cries, blood and something white sticky, someone stands and looks at him, he thinks it's him. He's angry that he's crying. Then he sits in the locker room, his dad comes in to get him and asks if everything went well. He stares straight down at the bench, it's as if he's not there. He goes to the car, but he's just gone, he doesn't exist.

Journal entry woman SAIS 6 DID
The patient begins the session by saying that now I know that my mother knew what happened to me 100%. She came in once when I was 5 and my father raped me, she saw and left. The patient feels the betrayal.

Fight, Flight

Fight, flight, freeze, and fawn are our four primary responses when the body's sympathetic nervous system is under stress or danger. Trauma therapists define these reactions as a neurobiological response to threatening situations. According to Malchiodi (2020); referenced in Psychology Today, there is a universal understanding of the thinking brain (neo-cortex) which is often automatically dominated by our midbrain, specifically the amygdala which regulates fear and terror. This means that the midbrain goes on high alert and signals the sympathetic nervous system to release chemicals that prepare the body to flee or fight. However, flight is not possible when the limbic system engages the parasympathetic nervous system which initiates the freeze or collapse response in the body which results in immobilization, restricted breathing, and decreased metabolism. The responses occur automatically and are deeply integrated within us humans and have aided in our survival. They are triggered from the amygdala, the part of the brain that is activated during fear and terror. The signals are there to prepare the body to react when there is a perceived threat. *Fight* involves a direct physical or verbal confrontation in which the individual addresses the perceived threat. *Flight involves* an attempt to escape from the perceived threat. According to polyvagal theory (a theory about how the autonomic nervous system regulates our physical, emotional and social reactions to stress), the individual will try their newest system first when stressed, to escape the threat. The person will first initiate social skills and if that does not reduce stress, we will initiate the fight/flight response. If that does not reduce the stress, the individual will initiate immobilization as a survival strategy. In the case of sexual violence, it is mainly freeze and fawn responses that are relevant.

Freeze

Freeze has previously been called collapse and involves immobility, an inability to respond to threatening situations or the individual dissociating in response to the threat, a temporary paralysis or shutdown, the body becoming rigid and unable to move, which is a normal survival instinct in dangerous situations. Although freeze is characterized by a frozen movement where motor functions are inhibited, it includes an increased heart rate, rapid breathing, muscle tension, high blood pressure and analgesia (pain relief or freedom from pain) that prepares for the fight/flight response (Van der Hart et al., 2004). Freezing to ice, becoming rigid or completely shutting down can prevent further damage when it is not possible to escape or fight. Unbearable, intense emotions become too overwhelming for the person to organize, take in information or think. In the animal kingdom, there are several examples of animals that play dead when they are caught by a predator. When an individual experiences freeze, the metabolism slows down, which makes the person feel less active. Dissociation occurs in freeze.

Journal entry woman SAIS 3

She describes being petrified during the assault and blames herself for not leaving.

Journal entry woman SAIS 5

The patient sells sex for money. He drives her to a parking lot, his eyes are changing, she goes into freeze mode and he orally rapes her by forcing his penis into her mouth. During the assault, she changes into a child part who is 5 years old, he calls her a whore, takes a stranglehold on her neck and says she wants to be raped. It is the 5-year-old part who appears in the therapy room and carries the memory of the rape.

Fawn

Fawn implies an attempt to please or not to resist, a total submission, to avoid conflict or danger. Taylor et al., (2000); referenced in Psychology Today coined the term "tend and befriend" as a stress response for women. Researchers suggest that tending (care or look after) was designed to protect themselves or their offspring and to befriending involved an establishment of social networks. The research team found that the flight response was not possible for some women and that providing care to try to influence their social survival functioned under stress. A few years later, fawn was added as a trauma response. The terminology comes from Walker (2003); referenced in Psychology Today who described fawn as *codependent defense* and continued in the footsteps of traumatology and chose to begin the new concept with the letter, F. Hence the four Fs in trauma psychology, Fight, Flight, Freeze, Fawn. Walker described fawn as the individual seeking safety and security by merging their needs, desires and wants with others, sometimes with the perpetrator. These individuals respond to stress and trauma by forfeiting their own rights and transgressing their own boundaries by becoming compliant and/or helpful.

Fawn is often the consequence of a long process of degradation where the opposite, resisting, is associated with enormous suffering. The perpetrators teach the victim that no matter how you move, you will stumble, go in circles and then come back to where you started. The degradation leads to a constant state of surrender. Fawn can also be described as a lack of one's own identity and limitlessness by becoming so overwhelmed that the individual cannot stand up for themselves. Words such as *people pleaser* or passivity, when they are subjected to assault, abuse or terror they suffer from the true meaning of the word fawn, they write down their own value, act derogatory, belittling, nonchalant and shame-based towards themselves.

A good exercise for patients who use fawn as a defense is the "No Exercise." The therapist should ask several questions and the patient can only answer no. Can you hand me a glass of water? *-No,* Could you be so kind as to take back what you were talking about before? *-No,* Would you like to tell me your last name? -The best. Can't you open the window a little, it's so hot in here? *-No,* etc. The exercise is to help the patient examine what feelings arise from denying, from saying no.

Journal entry woman SAIS 5
The patient has CPTSD after being locked up and abused by her perpetrator for over a year. He had locked her up and lent her out to other men as payment for debts in the criminal world. The patient described that she lived completely in the perpetrator's world of experience, he was on hard drugs, was a career criminal and raped her in hours-long assaults. She has visited the health care with major injuries to her genitals but has not been able to tell that she is being abused. She became co-dependent, took care of her perpetrator and was nice and compliant to those who guarded her. She was driven to work by the man's criminal friends, bruised, but like women who are victims of violence in intimate relationships, she never gave up her perpetrator when the employer asked. At the end of the relationship with her perpetrator, she has completely written off her own value and blames herself.

Journal entry woman SAIS 4
The patient has different ego-state parts, the little part that wants to do everything right (1-10 years), the shut-off whore, the rejected part, the kind part, the vulgar part and the docile part.

Gang rapes

In prolonged abuse where children have been exposed within pedophile circles and the infant or young child (up to 5 years) during the abuse goes from one arm to the other, severe dissociative injuries are formed. When the next arm, the next perpetrator has a new way of inflicting pain and injury, which causes the child to temporarily exit or wake up from their dissociation when the perpetrator is replaced, which makes these memories extremely painful for the adult patient to revisit. When the defense of dissociation during the abuse was put out of play.

Journal entry woman SAIS 5

The patient (5 years old) says that her father and another perpetrator take her to Turkey, she is drugged and put in the back seat of a car, at the border crossings they put her in the trunk. She remembers going on stage, several men booing in the audience, she is wearing pumps and a dress, she falls because she is so drugged. She remembers feeling sorry for the younger children who were going on stage after her. Afterwards she remembers that she is alone with a man in his underwear who is upset with her father and wants his money back because she is worthless, a fight breaks out and the men suddenly leave the venue. She thought they were angry because she fell.

Journal entry woman SAIS 6 DID

One part sees the situation from above, that the men are standing in line outside the room. They speak different languages, come into the room and pay her father. She leaves her body and sees the men on top of a small girl's body that is tied by the arms and legs to the bed frame, wounded, bleeding and pale. Between the abuses she comes back into her body and then dissociates again. The pain carries another part that we do not get in touch with, that part is called blue-red.

Journal entry woman SAIS 6 DID

The patient has been subjected to ritual sexual abuse as a teenager where the perpetrators had an infant with them. The part that remembers the abuse recounts the scene verbatim. She sends the following memory to for record keeping.

Only he can enter her vagina, the father says. Okay, right? Your turn, he says to a man standing to his right after he has finished raping her. Number two is a slim man with dark hair. A little tall. Don't come in her mouth, the father says. Okay, he says. He comes over the baby and stops puts his penis in her mouth and orally rapes her. Good job, says one. Let the father do it now, it's his daughter, he says in black. The father walks around and takes off his pants. He rapes the baby in the mouth and moans. Good, says one. Your turn, he says in black and points to the next man standing next to him. It just keeps going. It's so terrible. I can barely write anymore… I'm crying. It's so bad… Poor baby.

DID (Dissociative Identity Disorder)

DID arises after psychological trauma that started early in the child's life, is chronic and severe. A previous history of sexual abuse is found in the majority of all cases (Ross, 1989; referenced in Howell, 2011). DID means that two or more different parts within the patient have a common consciousness, a perceived place at the same time. One part may be aware of the presence of another part and have shared memories of the same situation, but this does not mean that they will behave as one person. Generally, one part is in control and another part or several parts are watching, listening and thinking about what is happening in a given situation. The treatment is based on achieving a common consciousness within the patient's system, which is a necessary step for harmony and being able to coexist as well as moving towards integration of parts (Howell, 2011). According to the National Institute for Health and Care Excellence (NICE) guidelines, there are currently no evidence-based guidelines for how to treat DID. The most common treatment is individual psychodynamic psychotherapy Brand, Classen, McNary & Zaveri, (2009); Putnam & Loewenstein, (1993); referenced in Rafaele, Huntejens, Marleen, Rijkeboer & Arnound, (2019). Medication and extensive psychotherapy are the main treatments. Although the disease cannot be treated with a specific medication, depressive periods, anxiety and psychosis are medicated (Yang, Luo, Liu and Wang, 2024). DID as a diagnosis is usually not made until the patient is an adult, long after the abuse that the patient was forced to endure is over (Lewis et al.,1997). According to Boon (2017), dissociative symptoms overlap with CPTSD and other dissociative diagnoses such as amnesia, problems with concentration and memory. Depersonalization, derealization and intrusive traumatic memories can also be intrusions from dissociative parts or voices. The difference is that in DID the parts are characterized and experienced as *not me* and in CPTSD the emotional stages are characterized as *I*. There are many factors that contribute to the misdiagnosis of DID. One is that DID patients rarely disclose their dissociative symptoms, avoiding reporting them unless directly asked. Because healthcare professionals are generally not trained to diagnose DID, the appropriate questions are rarely asked and the symptoms are never detected. This often results in clinicians opening up for a more familiar diagnosis such as schizophrenia or borderline (Cortez, 2022). Patients with severe trauma usually do not present their traumatic history as they do not want to connect their experiences of trauma with their current symptoms. When we talk about abuse that leads to DID, we mean extreme sexual abuse with torture-like elements where the perpetrators psychologically manipulate their victims to control their thoughts and behavior in the moment and in the long term. They may have a phobic attitude towards all emotions related to the trauma or have amnesia for parts or all of the trauma. Patients present with various symptoms such as mood problems, eating disorders, sleep problems, anxiety, alcohol and drug use, somatic, relational or sexual problems. According to Brandt et al., (2016), Borderline and DID are superficially similar with a similar psychological profile and symptom picture such as abrupt mood swings, identity disturbance, impulsivity, risk-taking behaviour, self-harm and suicide attempts. The DSM (Diagnostic and Statistical Manual of Mental Disorders) was created to ensure consistency and reliability in diagnosis by ensuring that all clinicians use the same language. In practice, all clinicians, even if they have never met a DID patient before, should be able to use the manual to give a correct diagnosis, but this is not the reality. Historically, the DID diagnosis has been dominated by adult women. The presence of amnesia has been reported since the first edition of the DSM, as well as the fact that symptoms begin and end suddenly, the word alternation first appeared in the third edition, later it was added that DID involves two or more subpersonalities within the same person APA, (1980), (2013); referenced in Cortez, (2022).

Of the various psychological difficulties or illnesses that can arise after trauma, DID is the most severe and most chronic. Dissociative symptoms are found in many psychiatric diagnoses, but the highest levels of dissociation are found in DID Lyssenko et al., (2018); referenced in Rafaele, Huntejens, Marleen, Rijkeboer & Arnound, (2019). Allison Miller chooses to speak of DID as a mental injury instead of a mental illness, because it is because someone has injured the patient that the illness has arisen. DID means that the patient has a disruption in the identity regarding the sense of a self and agency (ability to act and influence their environment) which forms changes in affects, behavior, consciousness, memory, perception, cognition and sensorimotor functions. In addition, the patient experiences memory gaps in everyday events or of important personal information/traumatic events (DSM-5; American Psychiatric Association, 2013). Dissociative injuries have a strong correlation with self-harm behaviors and multiple suicide attempts. DID patients have a high risk of early death and are the most costly patients in the health care system Galbraith & Neubauer, (2000); referenced in Rafaele, Huntejens, Marleen, Rijkeboer & Arnound, (2019). DID patients are often excluded from studies due to their complex poly-symptom picture and long treatment times. Many symptoms that DID patients experience are misunderstood within healthcare. In Schröder, Nick, Richter-Appelt and Brinken's study from (2018) where 165 participants self-estimated that they had been exposed to organized and ritual abuse, 69.1% reported that they had been misdiagnosed within healthcare at least once in their lives. The most frequent misdiagnoses were borderline personality disorder (43.9%), schizophrenia (21.1%), psychotic illnesses (22%). Which in turn results in incorrect medication, incorrect treatment and/or lack of treatment. Dissociative symptoms such as feelings of unreality and hearing voices coming from inside were examples of symptoms misinterpreted as psychotic or hallucinogenic. In Kloet et al., the study referenced in Yang, Luo, Lio, and Wang (2024), patients with DID scored higher than those with PTSD on fantasy tendencies, cognitive impairment, and sleep disturbances due to nightmares.

As a clinician, you need to be aware of subtle shifts in the patient. The shifts involve large gaps in autobiographical memory, logically inconsistent pieces of the narrative, a history of abuse, experiences of depersonalization or derealization, affective dysregulation, and somatoform dissociation. Large gaps in autobiographical memory and a history of abuse are red flags. For example, you can ask questions like "can you sometimes experience things that are not real?" or "can you sometimes feel like you are not in your body?" Patients with DID often believe that this is how everyone feels and do not see this as important information to share when making a diagnosis. You can also ask whether the patient has thoughts that are not perceived as their own. Chefetz (2000); referenced in Howell, (2011) describes how a patient responds when asked if she ever experiences other voices. "She looks confused and says - oh you mean my people, absolutely, they've been there as long as I can remember. How did you know?, no one has ever asked". Standard questions should include a) experienced parts within the patient, b) amnesia, c) PTSD symptoms and f) affective symptoms. In addition to these, the interview should include questions about memory and amnesia, experiences of derealisation and depersonalisation, identity confusion and identity shifts (Steinberg, Cicchetti, Buchanan, Hall & Rounsaville, 1993; referenced in Howell, 2011). One also needs to be aware of amnesia in the present, the patient experiences that she has "lost time", comes back to her consciousness and does not know where the lost time has gone. Does the patient remember what she did the morning or the evening before? Do you tend to buy things that you then do not remember, do not eat or wear clothes that you do not understand. A patient came home with clothes for a 13-year-old and did not understand why she, as an adult woman, had bought such small clothes. It is important to ask the patient what they remember from the previous session, as it may have been another part that was in the therapy room. There is also a benefit in asking which part was active during major events in the patient's life such as who got married, who gave birth, etc. The patient hears voices and in such cases the voices come from inside the patient's mind or outside the patient's head. This can be helpful in differentiating psychosis from dissociation Kluft, (1999); referenced in Howell (2011). To help diagnose dissociation there is *The Dissociative Experiences Scale (DES- II)* which is a form that takes about 20 minutes for the patient to fill out with various questions about dissociative states and events. There are also forms of *The Child Dissociative Checklist by* Putnam (1997), *The Somatoform Dissociation Questionnaire* and *Structured Clinical Interviews för DSM- IV Dissociative Disorder-Revised.*

To escape intense feelings of terror, constant flashbacks, a sense of needing to defend oneself, and poor self-regulation of affect, patients with DID often end up in eating disorders, substance abuse, sex as self-harm, severe masochistic problems that manifest in self-harming behavior (Howell, 2011). Brand (2011); referenced in Howell, (2011) states that suicide attempts and incidence (the number of cases of a disease that occurs in a certain population during a certain period of time) are 61-72% for DID patients. Completed suicides are found in 1 to 2.1% of patients with DID.

Various multiple conditions have been described over time by several well-known theorists, such as Pierre Janet, Sigmund Freud, Alfred Binet, Enrico Morselli, and Sandor Ferenczi. Many of the patients diagnosed with hysteria in the 20th century would have been diagnosed with DID today. The current debate regarding the validity and etiology of DID echoes earlier debates about hysteria and other trauma-based phenomena such as dissociative amnesia. The previous lack of systematic evidence on the relationship between trauma and clinical symptomatology contributed to misconceptions regarding trauma-related problems (Brandt et al., 2016). Rosenbaum, cited in Brandt et al., (2016), argues that as the concept of schizophrenia became dominant among clinicians, the concept of DID declined significantly. In the new climate of receptivity (assimilation of impressions) regarding studies of trauma, research on dissociation and DID has expanded rapidly between 1975-2015, research on dissociation and dissociative disorders exists all over the world (Brandt et al, 14,34,3,12,35-45; 2016)

Journal entry woman SAIS 6 DID
The patient is hospitalized for psychosis which was likely intense flashbacks.

Three phase therapy

According to the International Society for the Study of Trauma and Dissociation (ISSTD, 2011), treatment of DID is generally carried out based on three steps or phases and they believe that treatment must be holistic. The goal of treatment is to increase the degree of shared consciousness for the parts, communication and integrate and unite functions from different parts, which facilitates the processing of traumatic memories in order to integrate separate identities in the second and third phases of the therapy process. In the first phase, the therapist should create security and stabilize the patient's symptoms. In the second phase, the patient is exposed to traumatic memories that are confronted and processed. In the third phase, therapy is concluded through integration and psychoeducation. The trauma-focused phase should only be started when the patient has relatively few life stressors, sufficient ego strength, a commitment to treatment, social support, financial resources and other factors that help the patient undergo such a demanding treatment. Which few DID patients achieve. As a result, many patients stay in phase one throughout the treatment period. According to the ISSTD, traumatic incidents cause strong emotions, which makes DID patients more likely to act out both against themselves and others. As a result, therapy should focus on the violent tendencies that the patient shows, by receiving cognitive therapy in the initial phases to increase their impulse control. In the first initial part of therapy, the therapist should focus on stabilizing exercises, safety issues, symptom stabilization, and establishing a therapeutic alliance. If one fails to stabilize the patient and focuses too early on detailed exploration of traumatic memories, the patient's functions will deteriorate and the patient will have a reduced sense of security (Brandt et al., 2016). In addition, therapists need to be prepared for the fact that some patients do not want to synchronize and integrate their parts. As a therapist, one needs to be aware of how the patient's resistance manifests itself based on the degree of traumatization. In SAIS 1-2 the resistance looks like traditionally described with regression or dissociation, in SAIS 3-4 sub personalities (ego states) will emerge and in SAIS 5-6 protective parts of the patient will emerge. If you as a therapist choose to address the resistance, it needs to be presented with an empathetic and soft appearance to the patient, so that you can jointly explore where it originates from.

The trauma-focused phase is considered destabilizing for chronically low-functioning patients, including those with attachment problems, minimal ego strength and coping strategies, where the perpetrator is still active, major medical problems or addiction and dependence. The consequence of this is that many patients stay in phase one for a very long time, sometimes the entire treatment because the right conditions do not exist to move on to phase two. In the third phase, the material is integrated and the patient is rehabilitated. This is followed by the ability to regulate affects and manage the patient's symptoms, the patient begins a grieving process and resolves their traumas (Brandt et al., 2016). The goal is for the patient to gain increased awareness of themselves and their parts, an integrated sense of function between the parts and increased communication between them. If the therapist stays too short in the stabilizing and reassuring phase, there is a risk that the patient will become overwhelmed when the uncovering of memories begins and the symptoms worsen (Brand, Lowenstein & Spiegel, 2014). However, it is difficult to measure the effect of the therapy as the studies that have been conducted have been very small. When the patient's symptoms have decreased, it is difficult to measure what it is actually due to as the treatment period is so long, the placebo effect or alternatively just the passage of time etc. It is usually individual therapists who work with DID patients and they have their own methods, so it is the method or the therapist's skill that is measured.

As well as the difficulty as there are no groups to compare the results with and the high number of patients who drop out of studies. Brand et al., referenced in Brandt et al., (2016) has conducted one of the largest studies regarding the treatment of patients with DID (*N*= 230) patients and reported that after 30 months of treatment, the patients showed a reduction in dissociative, post-traumatic and depressive symptoms as well as a reduction in hospitalization, self-harm, substance abuse and psychological distress. The therapists in the study emphasized the importance of working with the sub-self in therapy, although they could not attribute the results entirely to working with the sub-self. Schröder, Nick, Richter-Appelt and Briken's study from (2018) which included 165 participants who all self-estimated that they had been exposed to organized and ritual sexual abuse as children reported that the abuse had lasted from birth to the age of 16. They became aware of their abuse on average at the age of 29. Awareness came for 76.4% as a flashback and for 66.1% in situations that triggered memories. Most reported that their birth family was a participant in the pedophile circle and most contained pseudo-ideological ritual motifs, or used dissociative split strategies such as mind control.

Cultural perspectives on DID

Although there is consensus that DID is a major health problem worldwide, there are major cultural differences in how the illness is expressed and how the symptoms are understood and interpreted within a cultural context. Interpretations are shaped by social norms in society, belief systems and historical traditions. Cultural differences influence how individuals experience their DID, how clinicians diagnose DID and how society perceives the diagnosis. The most common symptoms such as amnesia, depersonalisation, derealisation, identity confusion and identity shifts are universal but manifest from cultural perspectives. From being considered psychological fragmentation from a Western perspective to obsession in non-Western perspectives. This chapter will highlight interpretations of DID from North America, Europe, South Asia, East Asia, Africa and Latin America. By understanding cultural perspectives, clinicians and researchers can experience a more empathetic perspective, gain effective ways to approach diagnosis and treatment, and reduce stigma and improve outcomes for patients with DID Brand et al., (2016); Ahern et al., (2025): Nijenhuis et al., (1999) .

Western Perspectives: Psychological Fragmentation in North America and Europe

In North America, particularly in the United States and Canada, DID is framed within a biomedical psychiatric model, with multiple identities or parts, seen as internal psychological fragmentations resulting from trauma. Symptoms include apparent identity shifts, amnesia for daily activities, and emotional dysregulation often linked to childhood sexual abuse (reported in 90% of cases). The media portrays DID through television series such as *TheUnited States of Tara* or movies like *Split*, where exaggerated parts with distinguished depictions of dramatic behavioral shifts contrast with the often subtle clinical reality. This sensationalization fosters public misunderstanding, portraying DID as chaotic or violent, which can stigmatize patients and delay diagnosis. The individualistic culture emphasizes a single coherent self, making the fragmentation in DID appear as a strong pathological abnormality. Clinicians encounter patients who report inner voices or a sense of being controlled by alternative parts of the self, leading to misdiagnosis as affective disorder or psychosis due to the overlapping symptoms.

In Europe, DID is usually viewed through a psychological lens, but there are regional variations. In the Netherlands and Germany, clinicians emphasize somatoform dissociation as psychogenic (caused or exacerbated by psychological factors such as emotional, mental or behavioral states) non-epileptic seizures or loss of sensation, with studies reporting that 27-48% of primary care patients have dissociative symptoms. In England, the focus is on depersonalization with less emphasis on identity shifts, which is in line with a cultural restraint on emotional expression. Europe's blend of individual and collective values shapes DID as a trauma response. Historical spiritual traditions in southern Europe such as Italy and Spain may have influenced the narrative to include mystical elements. Stigma is less prominent than in North America, but with less awareness among the population and skepticism toward clinicians regarding the validity of DID, which contributes to underdiagnosis. European clinicians often require extensive training to be able to recognize the subtle presentations of DID, especially when the somatic symptoms are dominant.

South Asia: Possessed parts and spiritual narratives

In South Asia, including India and Pakistan, DID is frequently manifested as possession episodes, where the various identity states are perceived as external entities such as spirits, gods, or jinn (supernatural beings in Arabic and Islamic tradition). Symptoms include trance-like states, voice changes, and somatoform complaints such as gynecological problems or chronic pain that are culturally acceptable expressions of stress. For example, Indian patients may present with brief dissociative stupors (a state in which the patient is in a state of immobility and reduced responsiveness to stimuli) or report having shifted in their sleep, influenced by how local media portrays possession by a spirit. Collectivist cultures prioritize interdependence, where possession is viewed as a normal response to stress, often disconnected from a history of trauma. The spiritual framework reduces the stigma of dissociative representations but complicates psychiatric diagnosis as patients may seek religious healers or astrologers before seeing a healthcare professional. Clinicians working in these regions need to navigate spiritual beliefs, integrating them with a trauma-focused approach to avoid alienating patients Sar et al., (2014); Castillo, (1994); Shekhar et al., (2007).

East Asia: Somatic and masked presentations

In East Asia, such as China and Japan, DID is rarely diagnosed due to cultural stigma surrounding mental illness and the society's emphasis on emotional restraint. Symptoms are often masked as somatic complaints such as fatigue (a chronic and overwhelming tiredness), pain, or gastrointestinal (related to the stomach and intestines) difficulties, or depressive presentations that reflect socially acceptable ways of expressing stress. In Japan, as in North American countries, DID is frequently misdiagnosed as affective diagnoses due to subtle identity shifts. Chinese cultural norms, which discourage open discussion of trauma, obscure the possibility of seeing the origins of DID as patients present with amnesia (loss of memory or the ability to remember) or depersonalization that manifests after prolonged psychotherapy. Collectivist values prioritize group harmony, which prevents overt expressions of identity fragmentation (shifts) that further obscure DID. Patients often seek traditional healers, acupuncture, or herbal medicine before seeking psychiatric care, which delays diagnosis. A case study in China describes a DID patient who was initially diagnosed with depression, where the identity elements only emerged after a trauma-focused intervention, highlighting cultural masking (hiding one's features to fit in socially) of the core symptoms Xiao et al., (2006); Umesue et al., (1996); Kleinman (1986).

Africa: Ancestral Spirits and Social Acceptance

In African regions such as South Africa and Uganda, DID is often presented as possession by ancestral spirits or supernatural entities, with symptoms including hearing voices, trance states or alternate consciousnesses. In Uganda, experienced possession is something that mirrors DID with studies reporting severe psychoform (a mental or psychological dissociation in which thoughts, memories, emotions, behaviour and identity are separated from consciousness) and somatoform dissociation in 2-3% of women, often linked to trauma. Animism (the belief that everything in nature has a spiritual essence or soul) and spiritual beliefs frame the symptoms as socially normative, which reduces stigma but leads to underdiagnosis of DID. The patient's history of trauma is rarely acknowledged, with symptoms instead seen as internal psychological processes and not symptoms resulting from external forces. Traditional healers play a significant role, using rituals to address perceived spiritual causes, which can delay psychiatric intervention. Clinicians in these regions need to collaborate with cultural healers to create a bridge between spiritual and psychological frameworks, ensuring that trauma is addressed without dismissing the patient's beliefs Duijl et al., (2010); Swartz (1998); Van Duijl (2005).

Latin America: Syncretic Faith and Emotional Outbursts

In Latin America such as Puerto Rico and Argentina, DID is sometimes presented as nervous *breakdown* (attacks of nervousness) or as possessed parts, which mix psychological and spiritual elements. Syncretic means that it contains a mixture or synthesis of different philosophical, religious or cultural beliefs and practices. Symptoms include amnesia, identity shifts, fainting, psychogenic paralysis which are often triggered by stress or trauma. Patients in Puerto Rico may experience dissociative episodes during attacks with a history of trauma but then culturally masked. In Argentina, syncretic beliefs combine with Catholicism and indigenous traditions that shape dissociation into spiritual possession, especially in rural communities. Social oppressions, such as patriarchal structures, exacerbate dissociative symptoms, reflecting how cultural and systemic systems interact. The stigma surrounding mental illness leads to dependence on healers or family support, who often misunderstand dissociative symptoms as psychotic or neurological disorders. Clinicians need to navigate these syncretic approaches, integrating cultural rituals with trauma-focused therapy to address the underlying causes Lewis-Fernández et al., (2002); Guarnaccia et al., (1993); Ross et al., (2018).

Skepticism towards DID

Despite the fact that child sexual abuse is frighteningly common and stories of child abduction, sadistic sexual torture of young children are frequently reported in our news feeds, denial that child sexual abuse does not exist in our society is rampant (Howell, 2011). Denying the existence of organized child sexual abuse may be a way of coping with the anxiety that the realization of the reality would entail. One of the most frequent myths about DID is that it is iatrogenic, that is, something that has arisen or been influenced by the treatment or by the therapist. There are proponents who believe that there are several influences that affect DID such as suggestion (intentional psychological influence to change a person's way of thinking, emotional reactions and behavioral patterns), a tendency to fantasize, therapists asking leading questions, procedures and the media image of how DID is portrayed. Trauma researchers have continuously continued to try to challenge this myth (Brandt et al., 2016). The intensity of the memory war regarding patients who have told of ritual abuse and mind control has shown two difficulties in relation to disclosure. One is an empirical perspective (based on experience and observations) "is it true" and the other is a political perspective "what does it mean if it is true". The number of DID diagnoses skyrocketed in the early 1980s, with more people being diagnosed with DID between 1981-1986 than in the previous two decades (OpenEd CUNY; cited in Cortez, 2022). Some have suggested that the reason why a previously unknown diagnosis was now being identified so frequently had to do with sophisticated diagnostic techniques. Both interest in the diagnosis and the number of DID diagnoses declined during the 1990s, and it has been noted that the popularity was due to the film Sybil Paris, (2012); cited in Cortez, (2022).

In (1999) over 300 board-certified psychiatrists were surveyed, with 43% expressing skepticism about the DID diagnosis and 15% feeling that it should be removed from the DSM altogether, Gharaibeh, (2009); cited in Cortez, (2022). The DSM-IV describes DID as being particularly susceptible to suggestion, influence, and false memories that can emerge under hypnosis. Paris (2012) argues that because memories are narratives and not recordings, they are often not factually accurate and can therefore be altered and reinterpreted as they emerge. Many critics of the DID diagnosis describe it as an iatrogenic artifact created by narcissistic clinicians who desire the satisfaction that treating a patient with DID can bring. In addition, critics argue that the research comes from a handful of centers and that the research does not contain any randomized control to prove validity (Paris, 2012; referenced in Cortez, 2022).

DID in culture

Hollywood has shown great interest in the diagnosis of DID, although unfortunately the diagnosis in films and TV series has often been portrayed at the expense of individuals living with the diagnosis. Representations of DID are often stigmatizing, stereotypical and inaccurate (Snyder et al., 2024). Incorrect and negative portrayals of mental illness in the media shape viewers' perceptions of diagnoses and contribute to misconceptions and negative stigma (Coverdale et al., 2002; referenced in Snyder et al., 2024). Although DID is not an uncommon diagnosis, it is a hidden diagnosis. In contrast to how flamboyant or extravagant DID is often portrayed in culture, for example through the film Sybil starring Sally Fields, the transitions between different parts are often subtle or invisible to the observer (Petrie, 1976; referenced in Howell, 2011). Kluft, (2009); referenced in Howell, (2011) observes that only 6% of patients with DID showed clear alternations. The 1973 film Sybil is based on a true story about Sybil Mason who had multiple personality disorder (MPD) and was first published as a book that was later adapted into a film. One of the most recent films that portrays DID is Split which is about Kevin who has 23 different personalities that take turns coming to life and dominate the actions that Kevin performs. His different personalities work together to kidnap three girls for the 24th personality "The Beast" to consume. The film portrays

Kevin's different personalities as violent, destructive and cannibalistic which in short has nothing to do with DID at all (FAU Thrive, 2024).

Neurological insights into DID

Neuroimaging techniques such as structural magnetic resonance imaging (sMRI), functional MRI (fMRI), positron emission tomography (PET), and electroencephalography (EEG) have transformed our understanding of DID by revealing structural brain changes, functional alterations, and neural connectivity patterns that underlie its unique features. Findings shed light on the specific features of DID, such as identity shifts, dissociative amnesia, and trauma processing. This chapter brings together neuroimaging insights for clinicians, researchers, and students that highlight implications for diagnosis, treatment, and reducing stigma surrounding the diagnosis. Neuroimaging provides a universal basis for the phenomenology of DID, with cultural variations shaping its expression. Structural MRI studies demonstrate that hippocampus (a brain structure central to memory, learning, and emotion regulation) and amygdala (a part of the limbic system that plays a central role in processing emotions, particularly fear) volumes are reduced in DID (Vermetten, 2006). The reduction is linked to trauma-induced neurotoxicity (a toxic substance that damages the nervous system), while functional MRI (Magnetic Resonance Imaging) reveals frontolimbic (frontal lobe) dysregulation (inability to manage or regulate one's emotions) during identity transition. Biological markers, such as epigenetic (referring to inherited changes in gene expression that do not alter the genetic code, DNA sequence) changes, telomere (repeating DNA sequence at the ends of our chromosomes) ends and chronic inflammation, amplify these effects, together with cultural stressors exacerbating the psychological effects (Vinkers, 2015). In a Western context, identity transitions are psychological, while in South Asia or Africa they are spiritual, despite this the underlying neurobiological consequences remain.

Structural Changes: Trauma's Lasting Imprint on the Brain

Neuroimaging studies consistently identify structural changes in the brains of DID patients, reflecting the profound effects of chronic trauma on neurodevelopment. The hippocampus and amygdala, critical for memory consolidation and emotional processing, show significant volume reductions in DID patients compared to healthy controls. Research indicates that bilateral hippocampal volume is reduced by 15-25% and that the amygdala is reduced by 10-20%, likely due to the chronic stress-induced neurotoxicity from elevated cortisol levels. These changes are linked to the core symptoms of DID; a smaller hippocampus impairs memory integration, contributing to amnesia during identity transitions, while a reduced amygdala increases emotional reactivity to trauma-related triggers. A meta-study from (2021) confirms that hippocampal volume reductions are more pronounced in DID patients than in PTSD patients, highlighting the distinct neurobiological profile of DID (Reinink, 2021).

Cortical thinning is another hallmark, particularly in the medial prefrontal cortex (MPFC) and insula (a brain region that is altered in patients with anxiety), regions involved in emotional regulation and body awareness. MPFC thinning is associated with challenges in managing emotions, a common feature in DID patients, while insular changes correlate with altered body image, linked to depersonalization and derealization. Diffusion Tensor Imaging (DTI) studies reveal disrupted white matter integration in tracts such as the cerebral cortex and cingulum, which promote interhemispheric (between the two hemispheres of the brain) communication and emotional processing. Reduced connectivity (ability to be connected or communicate) in these areas may underlie the identity shifts in DID patients, as the brain struggles to integrate cognitive and emotional information across the regions Weiniger, (2013), Reink, (2021), Burez, (2019), Chalabi, (2015), Vermetten, (2006).

Functional Dynamics: The Neural Dance of Identity Shifts

Functional neuroimaging, particularly fMRI and PET, has revealed dynamic brain activity patterns in DID patients that offer insights into identity switching and trauma processing. Identity switching involves distinct activation in frontal limbic networks, including the mPFC, anterior cingulate cortex, and amygdala. During switching, trauma-related identities exhibit increased amygdala activity and reduced mPFC activity, which facilitates intense emotional suppression and daily functioning. These alternative patterns suggest that identity components serve as adaptive mechanisms, a compartmentalization of traumatic memories to protect against overwhelming stress and anxiety. For example, a trauma-related component may prioritize threat detection, while a neutral component may facilitate everyday routine tasks. FMRI studies have confirmed these patterns, distinguishing DID patients from control groups who have simulated the disorder, thus demonstrating biological validity of the disorder.

The default network (a network of brain structures that is active when you daydream), comprising the mPFC, posterior cingulate cortex (involved in cognitive functions such as memory, emotion regulation, and attention), and precuneus (involved in functions such as visuospatial imagery, episodic memory, and self-reflection), shows hyperconnectivity in DID patients when dormant parts are prominent. This exaggerated connectivity is associated with heightened self-referential (someone refers to themselves) processing, potentially underlying fragmented identities or deficits in autobiographical memory. Dissociation itself is linked to reduced insular activation (doing something active) which impairs the integration of bodily cues, contributing to depersonalization and derealization. These functional findings highlight the role of DID as a survival mechanism, where neural shifts enable coping with trauma, but destroy a sense of a coherent self Reinders, (2021), Lanius et al., (2010), Nicholson et al., (2020), Schlumpf et al., (2014), Brand et al., (2016).

Clinical implications: A bridge between research and practice

Neuroimaging findings have transformed the implications for DID diagnosis and treatment. Clinicians can leverage the findings to validate the biological basis of DID, counter skepticism, and improve diagnostic accuracy. For patients, understanding that DID as a diagnosis is neurologically based can reduce stigma and provide hope for healing. By integrating these insights into curricula, clinicians can better recognize subtle presentations of DID, such as amesia or depersonalization, and tailor treatments to address the neural impact of trauma. Culturally sensitive approaches are crucial, as DID's expression varies globally, from psychological fragmentation in Western settings to parts of non-Western regions.

Conclusions

As of May 2025, neuroimaging has illuminated the neural landscape of DID, revealing structural deficits and biological mechanisms that may underpin its unique features. From hippocampal volume deficits to frontal limbic dysregulation, these findings confirm DID's trauma-related origins and provide a robust framework for diagnosis and treatment. This scientific foundation paves the way for compassionate, effective treatment, reducing stigma, and promoting recovery for one of psychiatry's most complex disorders Vermetten, E., et al., (2006), Reinders, et al., (2015), Chalavi, et al., (2015), Nicholson, et al., (2020), Sar, et al., (2007), Brand, et al., (2016), Vinkers, et al., (2015), Dorahy, et al., (2014).

Parts

In cases of prolonged and extreme repeated threats, the self can also split and separate itself from its core self. Many with DID describe themselves as a *we* instead of one *I*. In the therapy room, the term "self" was used for the part that is present most of the time or the part that is usually present, or the part that is usually in control, but most often the word host part is used. Kluft, (1984); referenced in Howell, (2011) describes the host part as the part that has executive control over the body at most percent of the time during a given time span. The host part is often named the same as the patient herself. The host part functions as a front figure or as a shell for the patient. According to Lacter (2023), the psychological manipulations that the perpetrators use are systematic and dissociation-smart to induce and shape dissociative selves early in the child's life, often before the age of 5, when children are most sensitive to suggestion and trust adults and what they see and experience. Later, the perpetrators add several systematic strategies to enable the sub-self to function so that it serves the perpetrator's purpose. These strategies are called mind control and programming. The vast majority of DID patients have several child parts that are the parts that hold the most trauma memories, which is why they often find themselves in exile within the system (Schwartz, 1997; referenced in Howell, 2011) as the host part does not want to acknowledge their painful feelings (Van der Hart et al., 2006). Many child parts hold memories of terror, abuse and pain. Some may remain silent, while others whisper to avoid being heard or discovered. One patient describes her mutism as if someone had glued her lips together. Some child parts have the job of acting sexually (Howell, 2011). Patients may also name their shifts individually as, for example, coupling mode or that they are shifting.The self is created to protect the individual from the reality they have experienced. Rescue, comfort, and protective parts have different ways of manifesting themselves. Some parts can be overprotective in caring situations. They are often modeled after a real person or completely made up. Comforting parts are often adults like protective grandparents. They may have been named after someone who was kind to them in childhood (Howell, 2011).

Journal entry woman SAIS 6 DID

Pat has crocheted her inner reality and the different parts of herself have been given different colors. Before each session, she takes out the part that will be active during the session and the other crocheted parts of herself are put back in the cloth bag.

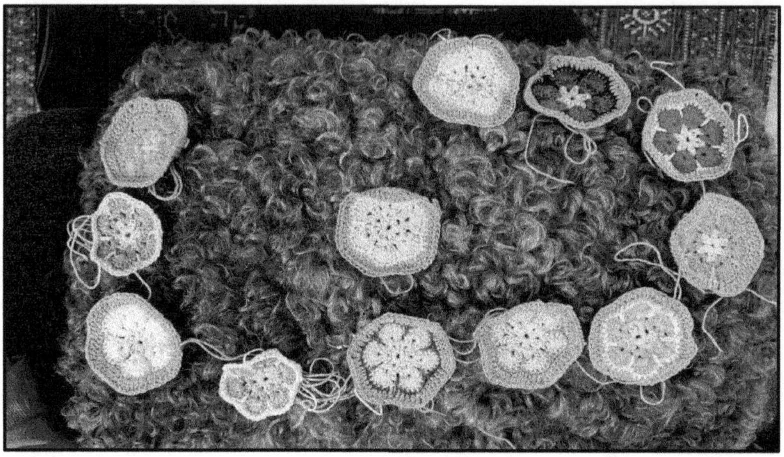

The number of sub-selves increases through the treatment as more parts emerge. There are approximately 2 years between the images.

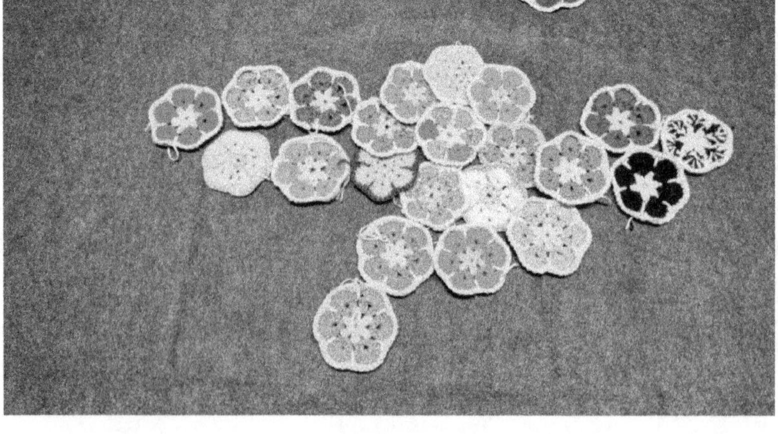

Journal entry woman SAIS 6 DID

The patient describes her inner space as a waiting room where all the younger parts want to emerge at the same time; she describes her host part as the now part.

Journal entry woman SAIS 6 DID

The patient describes that she has rebuilt herself into a whole external person who has arms and legs. The chest is hollow, where the shame is located, a neck, hips, mouth and eyes are missing. She describes that she feels patched together like a patchwork quilt.

Journal entry woman SAIS 5

The patient fluctuates in ability and some parts have high function. Through treatment, several parts have emerged that are not known to each other. There are very competent parts with also parts that are very small, with extremely low function level. DID gives an unpredictable rapidly fluctuating level of function.

Journal entry woman SAIS 6

During years of treatment, we have only had access to fragments of an assault inside a woodshed in the forest, we have followed the memory lane to the door and seen the backboard of the perpetrator who first enters and then switches to a part that lives through the assault but cannot talk about it. We have spoken to the part that is the one that leaves the woodshed but has not had access to the memory of the assault. During a session, we come into contact with an adult part that has been quite absent and only speaks English. I systematically ask which parts she knows and she replies that she knows the younger part that survived the assault in the woodshed well. When we ask the question in English and the small part is allowed to speak English, she can recount the entire sequence of events. Language became the bridge. Many patients remember their assaults in their original language, which can be an important key in trauma treatment to get hold of dissociated material.

Journal entry woman SAIS 6 DID

Right now, the competent part is there, but smaller parts cannot handle simple or multiple tasks.

Journal entry woman SAIS 5 DID
A younger part asks if I can adopt her.

Journal entry woman SAIS 6 DID
I tell the younger parts what year it is and that 30 years have passed since the abuse occurred. The 25-year-old and 23-year-old parts begin to discuss. The patient is allowed to think aloud in the therapy room. God, what has happened, that time has passed. Have you noticed that time has passed? one part says to the other.

Journal entry woman SAIS 4
The patient describes one of the parts of his ego-state as the protective (age less than 6 years) memorizing and reading all the details of his surroundings and what is said. Uncompromising, unyielding, lack of respect for authority, dry humor, never forgets.

Fawn or Feign parts

According to Malchiodi (2020); referenced in Psychology Today, parts of the patient can create adaptive coping mechanisms when faced with fear or threat. Fawning as a psychological response to trauma has been described earlier in the book while *feign* (pretending) is a complex strategy that the child learns in vulnerable situations to protect themselves. Feigning can be described as negotiating or improvising. Many patients describe how they negotiated with their abusers or pretended to respond in a certain way. We can also think of feigning as an important form of resistance. The child realizes quite quickly that they cannot escape or fight, so feigning may be the only way to influence their situation. To demonstrate resistance in feigning the therapist could use a more artistic expression when demonstrating resourcefulness, the action performed, which had a clear purpose of being able to influence one's situation, becomes an important part of the healing. You were cunning in gaining the trust of your perpetrators.The patient may have pretended to befriend their abuser, managed to postpone the assault, negotiated out of self-preservation or to save someone else. Patients have also described how they have consciously used (fight, flight, freeze) to become immobile, like animals that automatically play dead to escape predators. Malchiodi (2020) describes that patients can exhibit immobility not only in dissociative states but as a conscious and decisive action when they are in danger.

Faking is a determined action that helps the patient in the moment. However, the problem can arise when the patient has parts that are used to *people please,* negotiate, or befriending to survive and when the part becomes dominant. The part may value others more highly than the patient herself, find it difficult to describe feelings or communicate, feel abandoned or take excessive responsibility for others. It becomes crucial for the therapist to explain how these qualities helped the patient at the moment when they were in danger but that they no longer help the patient as a whole in the long term. This insight becomes especially important for the patient to exclude the shame that many survivors feel, blaming themselves for not using the fight or flight response in situations of abuse or terror.

Perpetrator parts

Within a DID system, some parts are likely to be perpetrator parts, which in traditional psychotherapy can be likened to identification with the aggressor or protective parts. Perpetrator parts generally hold rage and contempt towards the host part and they are often responsible for self-harm and may act suicidally towards other parts. They are often teenagers or angry children who want to experience a sense of power (Howell, 2011).These parts may be created through mind control or arise spontaneously through traumatic events. Perpetrator parts may often tell the patient to *shut up* or *be quiet, call her a liar* and say that certain events never happened. These parts have previously been called persecutory-protective parts or trauma-bonded parts, which try to protect the patient from the perpetrators by acting like a perpetrator. It is said that every persecutor is a misguided protector (Miller 2014). In treatment, we need to help the perpetrator parts express their contempt and show their fear in order to reduce its intense strength. In a DID system there are often managers which can tell about the structure of the system and dilemmas within the system. Generally, managers are affectless and give a mute impression (Putnam, 1989; referenced in Howell, 2011).

Many times, perpetrator parts are named after the devil, Satan, Lucifer (Kluft, 1994; referenced in Howell, 2011). Boon (2017) describes that the host part is often afraid of persecuting perpetrator parts and believes that their voices belong to external perpetrators. It is important to ask perpetrator parts what they have been through, show care and explain to the patient that at one time the part was needed to survive and we need to show respect. Perpetrator parts may also be afraid of the therapist as they do not want to give up their position of power, they may be worried that the therapist will never want to work with them. The perpetrator parts are a) lonely, b) hold the worst feelings of anger, shame and powerlessness, c) are terrified of crying, sadness or vulnerability, d) are terrified that they will disappear, e) have extremely bad feelings about themselves, f) believe that the therapist will never want to work with them, g) believe that they will either be destroyed by the therapist or destroy the therapist, h) lack cognition about healthy independence. Here Boon means that the therapist needs to assure the perpetrator parts that they are important parts of the self, they will not disappear, they can find other ways to deal with feelings of anger, rage and powerlessness, they can maintain control even if they work with the therapist. They will not appear weak or frail because they work with the therapist and they are not losers if they cry or show vulnerability. It is only when the therapist deeply understands the psychological power of the perpetrator parts created through mind control that survivors can reveal themselves and tell that they have been subjected to forced abuse. Forced to commit abuse against other innocent animals and children. Persecuting parts often punish other parts for various things, such as telling someone about the abuse, which the perpetrator said needs to remain a secret or for other activities that were forbidden in childhood (Howell, 2011).That the patient has parts whose function is to harm others, how they condemn themselves and the moral damage they feel because of the abuse they have been subjected to. They are worried that the therapist will condemn them, it is only when the therapist understands them and their complex systems that we can help them find self-care and share their grief (Lacter, 2022).

Parts within a DID system often have different genders with stereotypical expressions (Howell, 2011). Lewis et al., (1997) conducted 12 (11 men and 1 woman) interviews with people convicted of murder with a DSM-IV DID diagnosis. Their dissociative symptoms were categorized as; trance-like states, amnesia for long periods, peculiar behaviors, changes in voice and demeanor, and auditory hallucinations. The trance-like states they described had also been observed during the interviews. The participants described it as if they had been in astral projection at the time of the murder, that it went blank, "spacing out," or that they were transported to imaginary places in their heads, seven of them admitted that they could block out all forms of physical pain. All 12 participants had voice and behavior changes, one woman switched to an aggressive man and other men switched to women. One participant did not recognize his own voice from another part of the courtroom and all 12 participants had used different names on different occasions, although not in the context of escaping arrest or responsibility. Ten of the participants had markedly different handwriting and signatures on different occasions. Nine of the participants, including the female participant, had violent male parts that most described as taking all the pain. Six of the participants had older female parts whose function was to care for, comfort and protect. The majority of the participants had parts that represented abusive fathers, mothers and other relatives. According to Lewis et al., (1997) the term abuse is not accurate to describe what the participants had suffered as children and they use the word torture as a better descriptive term. They mentioned examples of one participant having been set on fire by his parents, one having been exploited in child pornography by his stepfather and having severe injuries to his anus after being forced to sit on a hot plate. Another participant had had his penis scalded when his father tried to circumcise him and another had been tied up by his mother and forced to drink blood and had tampons inserted into his anus to simulate menstruation. The authors were surprised that none of the participants had raised childhood abuse as a mitigating circumstance in the courtroom and that their hosts minimized and denied that they had been sexually or physically abused.

When specific dissociative parts within victims of extreme sexual abuse act out through violence, the rest of the system may experience it as "losing time". According to Groth (1979); referenced in Lacter (2022), this type of amnesia is called "red-outs". Groth argues that most of the literature on violent offenders and psychopathy neglects how childhood sexual abuse affects the etiology (the doctrine of cause and origin). When violent offenders act out, it is missed that dissociated parts so-called "red-outs" may be dissociative parts that are the ones who carry out the crime. According to Lacter (2022), victims of extreme sexual abuse rarely become violent offenders, but that violent offenders are almost always victims of severe abuse and that our legal system misses that many of them have DID.

Journal entry woman SAIS 6 DID
The woman has a mute part that exposes the system to self-harm. I can only speak to the part via writing, we chat during the sessions in an app. The part has been told that she is not allowed to tell anyone, but chatting is not classed as telling. The concept did not exist when the memory was encoded.

Journal entry woman SAIS 5
The patient has a part of her that is suicidal and self-harms by swallowing razor blades, batteries and hanging herself. It is the perpetrators who have told her that she should die that has been internalized into a part that attacks the body. The voice says that she must harm herself and it is not possible to negotiate with that voice. She also has a part that wants to be taken care of and not have to take any responsibility after the self-harm and suicide attempts. She has a part that wants to die and a part that wants to live.

Journal entry woman SAIS 5 DID
The voice tells her to get a knife, it sounds dull and not like her own voice. She has a flashback that she has blood on her hands, she sees him standing there looking at her, he is a shadowy figure.

Journal entry woman SAIS 6 DID
The voice is melodious but he rules in the background.

Somatoform Dissociation

Somatoform dissociation is a condition in which bodily (somatic) functions, such as pain, movement, or senses (sight, hearing), are caused by a psychological process with no identifiable physical cause. It is a form of dissociation or a lack of integration of bodily experiences. Patients with DID may experience themselves as different people, even as if the different parts have different bodies (Howell, 2011). Symptoms may include false pain, loss of pain sensation, or impaired movement. Physical symptoms without a medical explanation may be that the patient experiences actual physical symptoms, but there is no underlying medical or neurological cause. Somatoform dissociation involves a lack of connection between the psyche and the body, where the body's experiences are not integrated normally into consciousness. The symptoms may resemble neurological problems, but are called pseudo-neurological because they are not directly caused by damage to the nervous system. Common symptoms are pain, some experience sudden, unexplained pain, while others may lose the feeling of pain completely. Movement, difficulty moving the body or parts of the body. The senses, loss of vision or hearing. Other symptoms may be sweating, nausea or seizures that do not have a physical cause.

Somatoform dissociation refers to disorders that present with healthy symptoms, suggesting a general medical condition, but that cannot be fully explained by another medical condition, medication effect, or other mental health condition. Somatoform dissociation is often related to traumatic experiences, especially childhood sexual abuse, as well as cumulative trauma and threats to the body Sack, Lahmann, Jaeger, Henningsen, (2007); referenced in Schröder, Nick, Richter-Appelt, and Briken, (2018). Positive symptoms of somatoform dissociation are the "presence" of something new or changed, such as motor inhibition or anesthesia (loss of sensation), while negative symptoms are the "absence" of something normal, such as memory loss or decreased social interaction. Positive symptoms include physical "exaggerations" such as not being able to move or feel pain, while negative symptoms include losses such as memory lapses, feelings of alienation, negative mood, decreased activity, and a feeling of being separated from the outside world. The negative symptoms of somatoform dissociation can be converted symptoms such as loss of hearing, vision, speech, smell, taste, strength in arms or legs, paralysis, loss of sensations, emotions, hunger, pain, thirst, temperature. You are just a head, not connected to your body. The positive symptoms can be pain, tics, involuntary movements, pseudo-epileptic seizures, sensory perception, somatic intrusions, a feeling that your legs are moving but you are not moving them (Boon, 2017).

Journal entry woman SAIS 6 DID

Sometimes I don't recognize my reflection in the mirror, sometimes it and my body image change.

Journal entry woman SAIS 6 DID
The patient has emerged from another catatonic/stuporous state, now positive and curious. In a stupor or catatonic state, the patient is in need of full care, including being fed, helped to drink, shower, etc.

Journal entry woman SAIS 6 DID
We listen to the audio recording together and the patient gets carried away, vomits and becomes dizzy.

Journal entry woman SAIS 6 DID
Mental status, motor somewhat anxious. Slightly flattened facial expressions.

Journal entry woman SAIS 5 DID
The patient has reflected on when she goes into deep stupor states. There is an intellectual thought of leaving the body and never coming back. There is a pleasure in that moment.

Journal entry woman SAIS 4
The patient becomes highly activated during the trauma session and falls below the tolerance window, her body begins to shake and she feels it radiating from the uterus.

Constructed DID

Mind Control

According to Miller (2014), organized perpetrator groups have observed and studied for centuries how extreme childhood trauma, such as accidents, deaths, wars, natural disasters, repeated hospitalizations, surgeries, and most commonly sexual abuse, causes dissociation in parts of the child's mind. In the 1920s at the beginning of Nazism, organized groups developed ways to harm children and deliberately structure their victims' minds so that they would not remember what had happened or distrust their own memories. The consequence is that the memories become hidden inside the parts. Children's naturally occurring, adaptive defense responses that arise in the event of extreme sexual abuse form dissociative sub-egos. When a child is exposed to extreme sexual abuse, dissociative sub-egos are formed organically when the psychological and physical strain had become too much for any conscious mind to bear. The perpetrators use psychological manipulation of the child's sub-ego, which creates psychological mechanisms that control the victim over time. The perpetrators cause the child so much harm as to induce multiple dissociated sub-egos. They also create sub-egos that can continue to function outwardly, serving the agenda of the perpetrator network. Parts whose task is to keep parts separate. The parts usually know no other life than the functions for which they were created (Lacter, 2014). In organized and ritual abuse of children, mind control is a tool that the perpetrators use to gain control over their victims and their parts. Often, the perpetrators design memories that will cover up the original memory, which are impossible stories, such as being kidnapped by aliens. These memories are designed so that they will come up if the victim is asked about the abuse, so that no one believes them. There are also training rituals, such as the perpetrators saying that this is not real, this is a dream, at the same time as the abuse is taking place. Many survivors feel that they would have believed their own memories if only they had some evidence.

According to Gould, Cozolino, (1992); referenced in Schröder, Nick, Richter-Appelt and Briken, (2018) leaving the organization can lead to increased trauma-related symptoms instead of a decrease. This is based on the fact that in mind control the child has been programmed with techniques and parts that have an important role in keeping the victim in check so that they do not leave the group or expose its representatives. Mind control is complicated and different groups do different things. What is important for the patient is to come to terms with what has been done to them. Some can hold on to the images while others hold on to the sound. Mind control is created by a naturally reactive dissociative fragmentation caused by childhood trauma. The fragmentation occurs in early childhood and is often the result of life-threatening trauma. Dividing oneself is not something that the person chooses and it is not something that can be done in adulthood. Personality systems that are structured by perpetrators in groups tend to be better organized than those that arise spontaneously. The structured systems often contain a hierarchical organization where the therapist needs to get to know the leaders as all parts are afraid of them as they are the ones who threaten with tangible punishment. The process means that the patient's internal system needs to go from a dictatorship to a democracy which takes time and the therapist needs to be patient (Miller, 2014). Spontaneous DID is often more disoriented and unstructured in nature, patients with spontaneous DID are experienced as messy and unclear and often change frequently in the therapy room. In spontaneous DID, severe neglect, sexual abuse, often many perpetrators, several different ACE's have been intertwined during childhood, but in a more incoherent and chaotic structure. In the countertransference, the therapist can feel overwhelmed, everything feels fused and chaotic, often the patient lives in insecurity in the present.

There are mechanisms in extreme sexual abuse that can cause the child to continue their sexual victimization into adulthood. When the child is small, the perpetrators design the child to have parts of themselves that are extremely eroticized. They train the child to masturbate, be sexually abused, raped, sold, to produce film material for child pornography, etc. During the training, the perpetrators often provide the children with drugs that increase sexual stimulation or turn off pain. They reward the parts of themselves that demonstrate pleasure and torture and punish the parts that fail to show a sexual response. The parts of themselves do not know anything other than what they were designed to. One patient told me that during rapes she had cocaine injected into her vagina to experience powerful physical sensations, which led to orgasm during the rape.

Journal entry man SAIS 6 DID

The patient describes mind control via drugs as if they are implanting new information that the abuse did not happen. He describes it as if you are replacing the picture in the slideshow. A basement, he is 5 years old, different songs are connected to different events. A group of men hums, dark, a room, they have torture equipment, he is naked and hung on the wall with his arms up. He is given a powder and his lips go numb. He has to solve problems that are on the walls. They write things on the wall, he has to solve them in the meantime. He is punished if he does not pass the test, they pull his arms and legs, he faints from the pain. During the session, he paints in a block at the same time as the memory embroiders itself, in the picture a cage with a girl in it appears. He talks to himself, several parts want to come forward. There is another child in the cage, not him.

Journal entry woman SAIS 6 DID

The patient has sent the memory of some parts that remember a heart compression after her heart stopped when the perpetrators drugged her and filled her lungs with water. She writes down the scene with sound and image. They lay me on my back. "What are we going to do?" I'm lying on the floor. Nausea. Really bad. Breathing... Time passes... Just listen... "She's disappearing. Help here!" Says one. "What are we going to do?" Says another. "Wait here", says one. A person does CPR on me. On the left side and one blows three breaths. "Here she comes", says one. "Now we were afraid of you", says one. "Come and lie down." Is put in bed. "Are you okay?" "We're going home." "Wait a minute. We can just take some pictures", says one. "We're going home", says another. "Then it's just us here. We'll let her lie here", says one.

Journal entry woman SAIS 6 DID

They teach her French. She is 5 years old, naked, strapped in with an iron mask on her head, iron wires and electric shocks. Say meow, they laugh. Something heavy is placed on her chest. They call it a gift. The patient sends a picture.

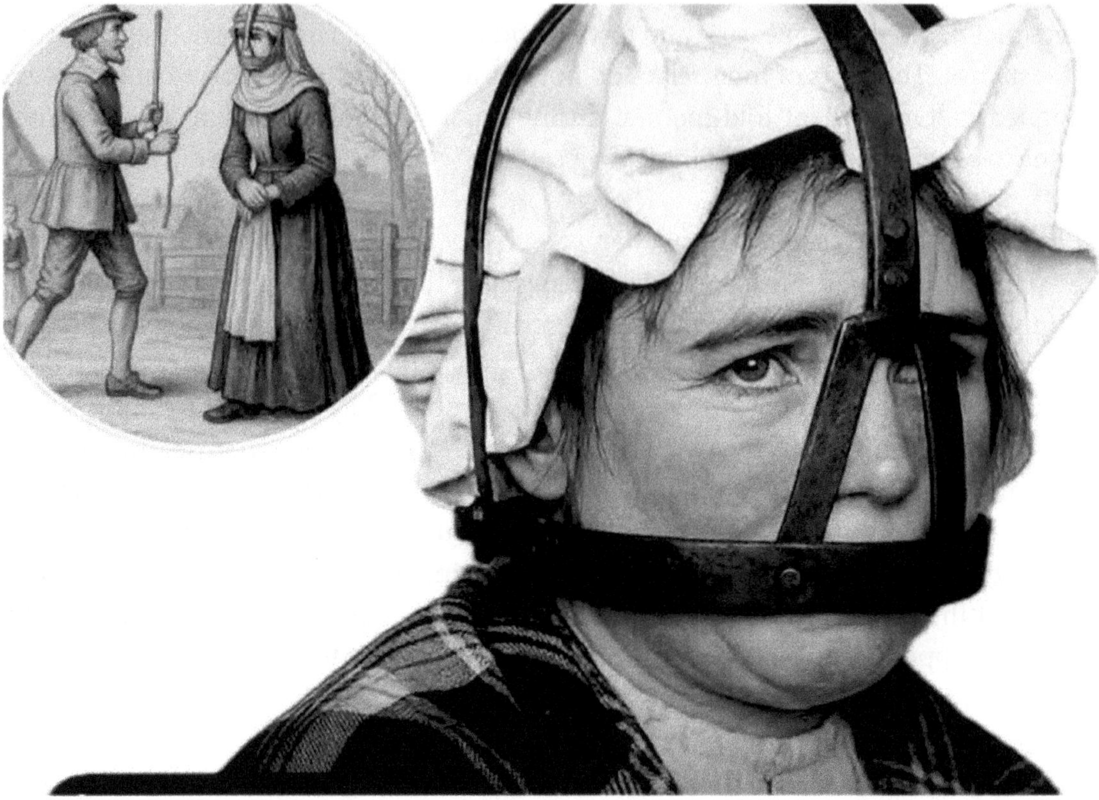

Programming

Perpetrators program systems and learning that will function as workhorses, Miller (2014) calls it Trojan horses planted by the perpetrators. They are often installed using suggestive hypnosis. Mind control is achieved through systems such as brainwashing, programming, indoctrination, hypnosis and with the help of drugs. The workhorses that have been planted are then used to *bleed through to* the host part in order to maintain control and submission over the victim in the long term (Lacter, 2022). Formal programming includes several mind control strategies to construct an internal landscape within the victim with multiple dissociative sub-selves in order to control the relationship between them (Lacter, 2014). Part of the programming is to achieve a moral injury within the patient. When something goes against the victim's moral assumptions. A moral injury occurs when (a) there has been a betrayal of what is considered right; (b) either via a person with legitimate authority, or by one's own "I did it" in high-stakes situations. Both forms of moral injury affect the ability to trust and create despair, suicidality and self-harming behavior (Litz, Maguen, Nash, et al; referenced in Shay 2014). A moral injury can occur when a military person performs an action in a war that goes against their own ideals, ethics or attachments (Shay, 2014). Within programming, several outdated dissociation-creating techniques are used that are still reported by my patients such as simulated drowning, being buried alive, filling the lungs with water, spinning the patient on a spinning wheel, spinning the child while looking up, shaking the patient to break the dissociation, etc. Many of my patients have become pregnant multiple times in their childhood and adolescence during abuse and fetuses have been aborted during ceremonies in various settings, many networks have access to medically knowledgeable participants.

Journal entry woman SAIS 6 DID

The patient is in a long memory lane with sadistic memories in a basement. They punish with words. They are organized, they have a pattern like a chain reaction, some do it in certain ways.

Journal entry woman SAIS 5

I am sitting in a bathtub. The film camera on a tripod is on the other side of the bathroom. The man is pushing me and my head under the water. I am forced to breathe water into my lungs. The water is flowing into the bathtub. He is pushing me forward to get the water out. I hear water flowing down the drain. Pain in the left side of my jaw. I am facing the rest of the bathroom. I am drugged and cannot resist. I cannot cough properly because I am numb/drugged.

Journal entry woman SAIS 6

The patient has had severe menstrual cramps which have led to flashbacks. She is in her parents' bedroom, she is in a part that sees the scene from above, something comes out, they have used something silvery, like forceps to pull something out. Grandpa does it, it is to be put in, twisted and it reminds her of when she was at the gynecologist, the cold feeling. They get something out, it is a small baby, it is a boy, she understood when she was standing in the shower. It is developed, a hint of when he turned his head, she could see a nose, lips and contours of the face and that it was beautiful. Previously during menstruation she has fainted or gone numb. They take pictures of her and the fetus, she is placed against a wall, she is to hold the fetus, before and after picture.

Journal entry woman SAIS 6
The patient sends her diary entries to U.S.

Living dead, or just dead, in a shell that I happened to be born in, I hate my life. Everything about it, because it's not mine, I'm not mine, I'm always someone else's. The senses are not mine, they must have had a thorough mapping to be sure that they affect all the senses and can destroy and restructure the brain and the thought patterns that they have created.

Strategies perpetrators use to achieve sub-ego

Dr. Ellen Lacter has worked as a psychotherapist in the United States for 30 years with victims of extreme sadistic, ritualistic, torture-based and mind control abuse of children. She has compiled the various methods that abuser networks use to achieve dissociative sub-egos within the child. She describes that the therapist needs to have knowledge of how mind control works in order to help patients overcome its harmful effects.

Conditioning- operant, classical, fear conditioning

Conditioning involves putting the child in a suitable state for a certain purpose and operant is the learning process that is carried out where the consequence of a certain action results in a reward for the child. Conditioning is the most common way to control the victim's thoughts and behaviors, thus the most common approach to achieving mind control. It includes abuse and torture. The perpetrators punish and reward to control thoughts and behaviors. One of my patients was given the choice of a puppy that later was to be killed. A patient told me that she was given the opportunity to raise baby rabbits whose skins the father later nailed to a plank in the garage and the meat was served for dinner.

Journal entry woman SAIS 6 DID
Pain should be pleasure, my body is like rubber, I don't want to see, I remember the pain.

Fear conditioning

Using fear and terror is a classic way to pair different stimuli. For example, the perpetrators can play a certain song while torturing the child. Later, the perpetrators can use the child's flashbacks and only need to play the song for the child to relive the torture. A patient goes into complete dissociation when a Latin song is played and cannot move from fear.

Journal entry woman SAIS 6 DID
The patient sends a memory:

"Now we're filming," one says. No! Help. Don't do that. No. Hold her, no, this won't work." I try to resist. "Get the rifle," one says. A man comes with the rifle, he aims it at me. "Now you do as we say," the man says. "Give it to me," another says. He comes all the way with it. It "Clicks." He took off the safety. Presses it into my left cheek. His head moves to the right. "Exactly, now you relax completely." He holds the rifle to my cheek. Doesn't want to. Help. Laughing. Terrified. Stomach ache. Nausea. Almost throwing up. Help. Fainting. "Now it happened again." "Get water." "Just leave her there." "Now we're filming."

Journal entry woman SAIS 5 DID
We're not done with you yet, if you think so. We've only just begun.

Journal entry woman SAIS 5 DID
He aims at me from a little distance. "If you don't do as I say, I'll kill you. You don't say anything!" he says. He puts the gun back in the corner of the bedroom by the door.

Journal entry woman SAIS 5 DID
The patient sends a poem about an assault.

Hide in the ground, crawl here close. They want to slaughter you but I know you don't want to. Dig your feet in, just stand still. Stand for a minute, breathe in, breathe out. The water is lapping, that's the last thing now, lie down here next to it and look out. Wait for the grave and breathe so lightly, no one will see you sink so easily. Take a message through the tunnel my friend, say goodbye to everyone you've known.

Journal entry woman SAIS 6 DID
There are flickers, images as if they are inside the eyelids, facial features that she sees clearly. Electric shocks in the head, in the eyelids.

Journal entry woman SAIS 5 DID
The perpetrator holds her under her stomach in the swimming pool while he assaults her and pushes her head under the water. Some part watch the assault from the side of the pool.

Journal entry woman SAIS 6 DID
The patient writes to me in the morning that she is in her mute part that is not allowed to speak. We meet digitally anyway and develop a system where she is allowed to nod for "yes", turn her head for "no" and have a session where I am allowed to speak to the mute part for the first time. The part is afraid, has been told to be quiet, there is a higher system.

Fraud

Deception means that the perpetrators deceive the child with lies, tricks, projected images, films, holograms, scenes, actors, etc. We must remember that the most effective age to create a part-self within the patient is before the age of 6 when they are most sensitive to suggestion and dependence on adults and their surroundings. A patient was deceived that she was raped by her dog, they placed the dog above the patient's face and the perpetrators then raped her under the covers. It is important in the therapy room to demonstrate to the child parts how they have been deceived. The adult parts can understand and tell the child parts.

Journal entry woman SAIS 6 DID
We go through the memory by talking about it like a dream, then the part is allowed to tell without being punished.

Journal entry woman SAIS 5 DID
Sometimes you can be sitting in a cell without knowing that the door is open.

Hypnosis

Children are naturally suggestible, they believe what adults say and do. Torture creates a heightened awareness within the child through pain, where the perpetrator is the one who controls the setting, the abuse and the child's survival. Hypnosis is used to make the child believe that the perpetrator has magical powers and is in contact with malevolent gods. One patient says that the perpetrators simulated that a demon had flown through the room by stretching a rope and letting a doll with a sheet over it go over her head.

Forced abuse

Sadistic abusers derive pleasure from watching victims harm other victims. It physically and psychologically affects two victims at the same time. The victims who are supposed to inflict harm on others are forced to do so and are psychologically distraught by their actions. The recipient of the torture of the first victim is usually both psychologically abused and sexually exploited through forced abuse. Abusers typically pair two children who care deeply for each other, often siblings, to create the most heartbreaking experiences possible for both of them. Being forced to act as an abuser is also an effective form of mind control. The effects are immediate and long-lasting psychological, morally damaging, creating self-hatred and self-blame. The design makes the victim feel complicit, unworthy of approaching anyone outside the abuser's group. It is an effective way to silence the child so that they do not tell about the abuse, expose the abuser, or seek help. The goal of forcing children to become perpetrators is to create dissociated parts within the child that believe they have harmed or killed others of their own free will.

Journal entry woman SAIS 6 DID

The patient writes to me about a ritual rape that she and her daughter were subjected to. She has been drugged and the father of the patient's daughter is the one who invited various perpetrators.

What are we going to do this time, he says. Take both of them to bed. We have to get them both. Lay her next to her. Put your arm out there. I'm lying closest to the door in bed. They put the baby next to me. She's in full force. They're chatting with her and she's babbling. Have you seen this before, a man says, showing her his penis hanging down. Are you filming? he asks.

Identification with aggressor

Identifying with the aggressor is a natural adaptive defense mechanism that arises when one experiences unbearable feelings of helplessness, terror, and feelings of annihilation that victims experience when they are exposed to extreme sexual abuse. In Stockholm Syndrome, the victim feels empathy for their abuser and by identifying with the aggressor, the victim wants to gain access to the abuser's power. The abuser can project their feelings during an assault onto the victim who, before separating themselves from the projection, may believe that they are the victim's own feelings. Our mind naturally wants to be a *top dog* and and get the experience of being an *under-dog* undone. The child internalizes the behavior of the perpetrator and identifies with the perpetrator's mind. Based on this, children can identify with the person who had control and power at the time of the abuse. Marvasti (1993); referenced in Lacter (2022) writes in an article about children who are exposed to extreme sexual abuse and post-traumatic play, that the rage and revenge reactions prevent the child from splitting their self during and after the traumatization. Hans Ulrich Gresh calls it "holy hate" which stores the righteous hatred and intense fantasies of revenge against their perpetrator unconsciously and in different parts of the self. It would have been far too dangerous to act out the hatred in conscious actions towards those who terrorize them during the abuse and often afterwards. In some cases, there may be an inevitable need for revenge that can be misdirected to safe and more vulnerable objects. For victims of extreme sexual abuse, the displaced hatred, the need for revenge and the violence are often directed at the self and other parts of the dissociative system sub-ego, resulting in self-harm or suicide. Many victims keep the dissociative parts that are born of rage separate from the other dissociative parts, other parts may be afraid of them and experience them as evil. In my experience, patients often hide the parts with hatred and rage long into treatment and the parts that have acted out against others often feel shame and guilt that make them unable or unwilling to come forward. One patient kept several sadistic mother parts that arose from torture by the mother confined until the end of treatment as they frightened the other child parts. Only when the child parts were treated and safe in the safe place did she dare to meet the mother parts and integrate them into the system. Usually, perpetrators who have abused other children are the last to emerge in therapy as they arouse immense feelings of sadness, shame, guilt and powerlessness.

Journal entry woman SAIS 6 DID

The patient has sent a picture of a skeleton where she has written about what the different vertebrae stand for. The skeleton under the blanket is my true self. Closeness equals violence, rape, every day is about survival. Gang rape equals my fault. A blow to the head. I deserve to be strangled and raped. I am there to be used for the needs of others, if I do wrong I will be punished. It is me that is wrong. I am waiting to die. I am evil, I exist to be punished. I am Satan's daughter, psychopath, pedophile, I am evil. I am a cheap whore, I only cost 20 SEK. A blow to the stomach. Blood, he laughs at my pain. My existence does not exist. I must deserve to exist. My body is there to be damaged, exploited and sold. If they punish me, they love me. I have to "work" to be accepted.

Journal entry woman SAIS 4

The patient was in her teens when she was subjected to an assault rape, after the rape she had high arousal, it felt like she had taken something, had a high libido and was hungry Primal.

Journal entry woman SAIS 6 DID

We focus on connecting with the parts that stay away or actively work to keep memories separate.

Deprivation of basic needs

Perpetrators create a systematic bond between themselves and different parts of the child. Usually they deprive the child of sustenance, touch, warmth, etc., sometimes until they are close to death. Then they subject the child to abuse where they have to agree to do unbearable things while telling the child that only I love you or that the perpetrator is the one who saved the child. One patient tells of day-long abuse by multiple perpetrators that the father sold her to. Some see the abuse from above as the men wait outside her bedroom in the hall for their turn. The father deprived her of water, rest, sleep, food, exposed her to multiple perpetrators. She has a part that sees from above a pale girl lying motionless in a bed. Another patient tells of a prolonged abuse in which she was locked in a cell and given no food for three days and forced to eat beetles and rats. The perpetrators were dressed up and wore black masks. Many of my patients have near-death experiences with various descriptions of light.

Journal entry woman SAIS 6 DID
He laughed at my pain, in the end the pain was the only thing I could feel and it was proof that I was alive.

Journal entry woman SAIS 5
She remembers that she needs to go through the memory to heal. There came the light, there she could stay for a while, a white light came towards her, a sound that is connected to it, birds chirping. A soothing sound that the patient likes.

Direct terrorization

Direct terrorization involves the perpetrator threatening the child to kill themselves or someone they love. A threat to kill someone the child loves can be an effective way to silence someone for decades.

Indoctrination into the perpetrators' beliefs or agenda

Many networks of perpetrators have political and/or spiritual ideologies. Some networks commit abuses in the belief that they can achieve immortality. Others simply use spiritual beliefs to intimidate their victims. Many of my patients have endured rituals where they have been reborn as Satan's daughter or have been married off to

Satan, who is often a man dressed in priestly robes and a mask. The ceremony often ends with the child (about 4-5 years old) being raped on some kind of altar in front of an audience.

Protracted abuse

In prolonged abuse, situations that last for days or weeks, often in cases of deprivation of liberty, different parts will carry different sequences or details of the abuse. Traumatic memories are interconnected and share association paths. When you begin treatment of a memory, related memories usually first emerge and then lead to other memories in the same memory path. How the linking looks differs between patients, it can be linked via the same time in the patient's life, for example a certain age, linked to a certain perpetrator, to a certain place where the abuse occurred, to a certain moment in an abuse. The patient initially does not remember the course of prolonged abuse narratively, or in the chronological order in which they occurred, but in sequences, disoriented memory paths, memory fragments and details. When you as a therapist work with a DID patient in the therapy room, we do not know whether we are working with a single abuse memory, a linked memory path or a prolonged abuse over several days. If we enter into a prolonged memory of abuse that lasts for several days, we do not know whether the flashback that has been the memory bridge is the beginning, the middle or the end of the abuse. As therapists we must accept that we do not know what we are entering into, this we share with DID patients whose parts have never before been allowed to emerge and the host part does not know what is to come. Svali (1996) referenced from www.endritualabuse.org, suggests that many survivors testify that their abusers subjected them to day-long torture where furious dissociated identities are formed. The child is beaten for a long period by a trainer, they are told to hit other children in the room or they themselves will have to endure more beatings. If a child refuses to hit someone else, the beating will be severe and so will the child they refused to hit. If the child still refuses or cries, the violent beatings will continue until they direct their anger at the other child. The steps are repeated until the child finally gives in and becomes submissive. Many times the abusers take the children to near-death experiences by burying them in coffins, hanging them on crosses, etc. They then ask the child "Where is your god now?". During long ritual abuse, the victims eventually become so terrorized and indoctrinated that they will do almost anything to function as a function of what the abusers want (Lacter, 2022).

Anneke Lucas, who herself was subjected to extreme ritual sexual abuse as a child and wrote the book Memoir of a Child Sex Slave (2022), describes a terrifying episode when her perpetrators tortured and terrorized her into, at the age of 11, killing another girl as "punishment" for sparing her own life. A sadistic way of robbing her of everything human and she describes how she thinks back and forth about the victim as a little innocent girl whom she does not want to harm and that she then sees her mother's face in front of her who sold her and abused her throughout her life. Lacter (2022) suggests that if she had not seen her mother's face on the girl, she would not have been able to complete the act, which she did. Anneke knew that if she did not do so, the act towards the girl's death would be horrific and prolonged. Protracted abuse almost always contains elements of multiple perpetrators and gang rape where the younger child is sent from arm to arm. The fact that the perpetrators are replaced affects the child's ability to dissociate from the situation, but they are often awakened back to the reality they want to protect themselves from. Many patients describe violent awakening attempts when the perpetrators try to break the dissociation through, for example, shaking and simulated drowning, we can interpret this as them wanting to experience the projection of fear in their victims.

Journal entry woman SAIS 6 DID

Pat is an adult woman with a constructed DID of about 1500 parts, SAIS 6 who has been exposed to incest throughout her childhood, sold as a child in a pedophile circle with ritual sadistic elements. When we enter the memory lane that will lead us into a three-day abuse situation she was exposed to as a 5-year-old, we have been meeting for 6 months in therapy. It begins with the patient writing an email to the therapist stating that she has become aware of how she is triggered by car doors, she describes it as being abducted. Each car door causes the patient to fall into fear and panic "I am being sold, hence all the doors. They talk about money and how much, there are many of them. I remember lying completely destroyed and apathetic as a 5-year-old". At the next week's session, the patient has had persistent dissociations and strong flashbacks, she begins to have memories of animals being tormented, suffocating screams of cats and dogs being raped and then killed. The different parts continue to write. An older part that is about 19-21 years old has emerged, which has meant that she has managed to do some household chores during the week. The patient writes that she feels that the flashbacks are starting to change in quality, they are in the same quantity and number as before, but now they are reconnected to where it hurts the most. A younger part that is present when she is 3,4,5,6,7,8,9,10 years old is confused and pushes forward, she has a sore throat, an adult part has long thought that she is allergic. The patient writes about many ritual details such as there were 13 poles, what they called those who were there, the animals, the cars that came and went, they gave her food, said it was a chicken but then turned out to be a cat and a dog. The patient feels an enormous care for the innocent animals, here she comes into contact with her anger. At the next session, the patient rests in a new part that has not previously emerged, she has changed her appearance and voice.

In the next session we go to a memory bridge from a fight between the father and a family friend, abuse and the patient sees the fight from above, she is sitting huddled on the floor in a corner. When we examine what happened before they fight. The memory of the fight connects in time after she returns from three days in the caravan. When asked if something happened in the caravan, an older, numb part enters and tells the story in general terms without any affect attached. I ask her to tell without emotion, only with sound and film, what does she see? We go through different sequences of rape and abuse, she has been beaten with kicks, thrown against a wall and beaten. Several men in the same clothes, ritual elements, they throw kittens against walls. They toast, drink, sing, clap hands. They tear animals apart and put the dog's head on sticks. They raped her in turns, individually and in groups, with a plastic bag over her head, anally, orally and vaginally throughout their stay. There are several caravans set up and other children, she remembers a 6-year-old boy. The adults argue with each other, someone gets upset because visible injuries are left on her. That was not the agreement.

When she switches to one of her host parts that has listened, she is shocked, she had no idea. We keep in touch over the next few days. The patient needs to rest but more sequences come up, more parts want to come forward. She describes it as if the memories are in a queue. She switches sharply in the next session, saying things, words that she herself does not understand. We go through the previous session and she feels confused because she does not remember what was said when another part was active. Afterwards, the patient sleeps for a day. She finds it scary to continue the trauma treatment and enter a trauma time when she does not know what will come up. She continues to write as more parts want to tell what they remember from the caravan "a boy is screaming - it hurts me - heartbreaking - helpless, someone is cutting him, he is still alive". Pat is completely exhausted from nightmares, new parts with memories that are in a queue and want to come forward. She feels relieved to send new memories by e-mail she can sort better. She writes that she remembers comforting another child by singing and putting a blanket over her. She quickly switches to a memory of being cold, naked in a pit. She feels cold earth, leaves, other naked cold bodies. They bury her alive, she gets earth in her mouth, can't breathe, sees a light. The memory lane transitions into total abandonment, naked in the caravan, in the forest, cold, hungry, tired, all her systems are completely activated or turned off. She wakes up on the floor of the caravan to a man lifting her up, tying her to a chair naked and raping her for what she believes is several hours. In other caravans there are other children, about 10, they don't let them meet. They cut her body, she sends pictures of the scars. After the session, the patient is completely exhausted and dissociates heavily. We will stay in touch during the coming day. She writes, panic attacks and death anxiety. She has difficulty thinking clearly or breathing. She writes that she feels constantly sick and changes 20-34 times a day. The pain is connected to a part that has not yet come forward. She feels numb. We need to go back into the caravan. She remembers how someone pulls her out of the ground, a tunnel approaching with light, first blurry and then a little more. She sees herself from above in the caravan, someone gives first aid. The body is lifeless and white. When I ask if she can see if her body has bruises or injuries, she says that it is another part that carries the black. More memories come from details about ceremonies, colors, symbols, what is said. Told literally, sentences that she, as a 5-year-old, does not understand. We help each other to interpret what they are saying and what it might mean in the vulnerable situation she is in. She draws what she sees and it is entered into the journal. The therapist becomes a witness. Now several sessions begin where she tells details, names and memories of prolonged rapes in and around the caravan, in other people's caravans and where other children are forced to participate. What clothes they want her to wear and unimaginable sadistic acts. The violence, sadism, ingenuity together with the perpetrators pushing the boundaries over the three days lead to the violence escalating and we note that not all the children came home. She was lucky to survive. In an almost surreal final scene where she sees everything from above in a dissociation she tells how everything is cleaned up, the participants thank each other in different languages, there is an organization, all the caravans drive away and the place is left clean, almost as if nothing had happened.

My patients have baptized various places as children and testify to prolonged abuse in caravans, the slaughterhouse, farms, incinerators, fishing, the king in the chair, initiations, tests to achieve various degrees.

Journal entry woman SAIS 6 DID
They put on a breathing mask with a tube so I can breathe. Lay me down in the grave. Feel the weight of what is being placed on me. The zippers of the body bag are pulled all the way to the pipe. Breathe. Drive. The car drives. There are two of us buried. As far as I know. A new car will be coming soon. They are obviously short on time, they have to do everything they have planned.

Organized and ritual sexual abuse of children

Since the 1980s, there has been evidence of organized and ritual sexual abuse of children through studies and documented material in pictures and films, as well as knowledge of how psychologically damaging it is for children who have been exposed. Organized and ritual sexual abuse of children is often rooted in the child's own family and generational incest is common, which is also associated with a higher degree of trauma-related symptoms. At the same time, critics have often denied that structured and ritual abuse of children often exists in the context of satanic groups or cults. The documentation, studies and experiences told by victims have been dismissed as the product of false memories. Children are born with the purpose of becoming a function of the organization and the pseudo-ideological content legalizes sexual violence. Survivors testify to occult groups that practice ritual sexual abuse of children, dressed in robes, torture and rape children in rituals, sacrifice animals and what the children have assumed were humans and celebrate the Black Mass. Sexual abuse of children carried out by a network of perpetrators who repeatedly and together prey on multiple victims is defined as organized abuse Salter, Richters, 2012; referenced in Schröder, Nick, Richter-Appelt and Briken, (2018). The tactics used by organized hidden groups are sophisticated, extreme and they are often invisible to the justice system and society, which makes them particularly dangerous and makes healing difficult for victims. In order to keep their existence secret, their members need to maintain normal lives on the outside. The perpetrators use various methods and techniques in the abuse, which are often based on ideological beliefs such as religious, denominations, religious orders, churches, etc. Occult societies often meet in groups of 13 adults, over 13 years of age and their children, on special occasions they meet in larger contexts (Miller, 2014). According to Salter, (2012); referenced in

Schröder, Nick, Richter-Appelt and Briken, (2018), the perpetrators use (pseudo)-ideological strategies with the aim of intimidating, humiliating and controlling their victims. They often use symbols, group activities with religious, magical or supernatural elements and force the victim/child to participate. By forcing the children to carry out horrific abuses on other children or animals, the perpetrators can cleanse themselves via exculpation, they escape responsibility through ritual abuse. Through rituals, the victims are indoctrinated into a violent and misogynistic worldview in order to control them. In Schröder, Nick, Richter-Appelt and Briken's study from (2018) where 165 participants self-estimated that they had been exposed to organized and ritual sexual abuse as children, approximately half of the participants reported that their perpetrators had a Satanist ideology (48.5%), a smaller proportion reported a religious ideology (19.4%), fascist (12.1%), racist (12.1%), and or right-wing extremist (8.5%) ideologies. Most of the participants reported that they themselves had been forced to use violence against other individuals (74.8%). Incest has a lot of research that shows that there are ritual elements in abuse that has occurred in groups. Many of my patients testify to sadistic gang rapes with multiple perpetrators and other children who were present as victims. Industrial areas, the order's villas, summer cottages, caravans, tent camps in the forest, apartments have been gathering points for pedophile circles with access to children. Today, child pornography testifies to pedophile circles that jointly practice sexual violence, sometimes with fatal consequences. Batiailles, (1994); referenced in Brunet, L., (2007) he describes the most central arguments regarding ritual orgies in the book *The Abscent of Myth* from (1994) when he relates the violation of the taboo to murder in war to the violation of the incest taboo during a ritual orgy. In both cases, Bataille describes the perpetrator's experience of tension and connection with the divine, sacred, or sovereignty of the natural masculine. He further described that a veteran returning from war can only experience ecstatic feelings by violating the incest taboo. The male initiation process generally demonstrates the ever-present threat that men and male relationships can pose to other men, whether in the trenches or the boardroom. A central ingredient of an initiation rite is that the initiate experiences vulnerability through the experience that marks the group's power over the individual. Once one has survived, one is in debt and is bound to protect the secret and is thus protected by the entire group. The cementation of male relationships occurs through terror, *We could have killed you but chose not to* Brunet (2007). Collectively, men take greater risks than they would on their own and the morale of the group is never higher than that of the individual group member with the lowest morale. In *Lambs Our Bodies Their Battlefield* there are no eyewitness accounts of men who tried to go against the group to stop the rapes or murders of the victims. The witnesses could always point out the man with the lowest morals who was the one who started it and other men who followed.

The ritual abusers harm the children by breaking the attachment relationship between the child and the mother, lack of care, terrorizing through costumes and coats, horror films, using blood, sexual abuse in orgies and rituals, sexual abuse by family members, using drugs, high-voltage electricity to body parts, punishment for disobedience through isolation, starvation, burial, psychological and sexual abuse and other forms of torture. Many times they simulate heaven and hell, force children to participate in sacrificial ceremonies, simulated cannibalism, etc. One patient says that when she turned 7 years old after being abused since birth, she was considered old enough and was allowed to participate in ritual abuse as a staff. Survivors of ritual abuse testified in Jerusalem (2025) about the abuse they were subjected to as children. Yael Shitrits said in her testimony in the Knesset (Israel's legislative assembly) *that you don't know what ritual abuse is, the human brain can't understand it. You can't understand what it means to program a three-year-old through rape and sadism. They can do whatever they want without anyone knowing anything about it.* She further describes that her trafficking took place all over the country, they moved her from ceremony to ceremony. Another survivor testifies that the ritual sexual abuse took place at public events and that there were internal ceremonies where she was handcuffed to a pole. She had to endure torture and starvation by well-known individuals in the community. There were ceremonial moments such as drinking menstrual blood and slaughtering cats and other animals. They had told her that no one would believe her if she told. There were ceremonies and rituals that were performed so that she would forget. She further claims that the police have known about this for years without being able to do anything about it because they lack the tools (The Jerusalem Post).

Journal entry woman SAIS 5
The patient is drugged and lies naked in the bathtub, unable to move. She sees the woman holding her newborn daughter and steps into the bathtub. The woman rapes the daughter while holding the baby's face up to the patient. The baby screams in pain and the patient cannot speak or comfort her child, she sinks into the water but is so drugged that her reflexes do not work. She gets water in her lungs. Someone pulls her up. They simulate that it is the patient who is raping her daughter, by placing the baby's face in front of the mother's. The perpetrators try to break the attachment relationship between the daughter and mother. Mom is disgusting, I will save you, says the woman. After the assault, they drown the patient. The patient only remembers the assault 25 years later when she has become a grandmother.

Journal entry woman SAIS 6 DID
They had a show where costumed children were auctioned off after dinner.

Journal entry woman SAIS 4
We are talking about the father's family, the grandfather has abused the brother and the father, the father's entire family belongs to white power and has a high level of violence and criminal activities.

Journal entry woman SAIS 5 DID
The patient has gained access to memories while drugged during the abuse. She sends every abuse she remembers.

7 rapes
Blood-filled stomach
Pregnant
Bird sacrificed
I am drugged.

A door opens. I hear someone come in. People are coming up the stairs to our house. They come in. In the hall. Have you given her anything. Yes, says A. I'm completely drugged. I don't know what to do. Take her to the living room, says one. I'm being carried by two. Carefully, says one. She's pregnant. They lay me down on something a little softer on the floor. In the living room. There's a ring of men around me. I recognize her, says one. She lived in X. They talk. Take off their pants. We're consecrating her to the devil, says one. One has a candle lit. It's white. They say hmmm. A pat (by chance or not, I don't know if it's part of the rituals). From earth you came, to earth you shall remain, they say. They pour earth on me. They hold a ball with chains over me and it gives off dust. They sacrifice a gray/black bird, I think. They smear something on my stomach. It is red blood. We dedicate this to you, says one of them, Satan. They clap their hands and press their stomachs. There is a trumpet instrument with who listens to the stomach on my upper left side. He takes the stomach between both hands and looks at it, what do we have here, he says. A beautiful baby. They laugh.

"We're looking forward to the baby," one of them says. He stands up. They walk around me in a circle. Who wants to go first says one. I want to go first, says one. He has an erect penis. Put on a condom. Be careful, she's pregnant. You see, he says. He puts something in my vagina. He rapes me in my vagina with his penis. My turn says another. He's taller than the first. He also puts on a condom and rapes me. Take the condom off afterwards. The third is a little thicker or rounder. He rapes me. Everyone is watching. Your turn, A, says one standing by my head. I can do it later, he says. No, now we're together, everyone has to do it for it to work, says one. A rapes me in the vagina with his penis. He doesn't have a condom on. My turn says the 5th. My turn says number 1. No, okay, then number one says. They did it in a circle, they started from the bottom and went up to the head and down again in order. It's clockwise when I see myself from above lying down. Last but not least, says No. 7 and laughs. A little more masculine voice, he's older. A little rounder. Big man. Put on the condom. There are seven of them in the ring. They pack up and get dressed. Take it, says one. You need it and give it to No. 6. Don't know what it is. No. 6 and one bathes me with lots of soap. Wash off the blood. Shower me with the shower head. Dry me off and put me in bed. They didn't wash my hair. They put my nightgown on and put the blanket over me.

See you next Wednesday, someone says. Bye. Bye. The front door closes again. A goes to the bathroom. I hear water. He goes to the living room/kitchen. Watch TV. Goes to the bathroom. Goes to bed.

Journal entry woman SAIS 6 DID

They lay me on the altar with my legs facing the exit. A man in black comes from the room where there is noise and he comes to the altar where I am lying. Who do we have here then he asks? What are we going to do here? What do you want us to do with her today? Can we sacrifice her? he asks in black. No, says C No? Okay, he says in black. It is as if he is whispering in the ear of the man in black. Yes, he says in black, yes, we can do that. Everyone stands up, he says. Everyone in the hall stands up. Come forward. They come forward. Put on your masks. They put on masks. Who wants to go first? he asks. I say one. Then you can consecrate her today, he says. I ask him. From earth you came to earth, you will stay. He swings over that ball with chains and dust in it that they have in the Catholic church. Where is the animal? Here, says a man. It is something brown with fur. Some oblong animal. It moves. You have to hold, he says. The man in black cuts the animal. The blood runs down my body. Then we will consecrate her to Satan. They smear me with blood.

Journal entry woman SAIS 6 DID

Of all the things we've talked about, there are 10 more systems. They are similar to the system that has been uncovered, with fragmentation and different memory paths, different traumas. The patient doesn't know what they contain, she thinks it's child pornography. They are behind each other so they are all their own, but they belong together. If the first container broke, there are several in a row. Similar but there is something completely different in them. They have always been completely closed. There is about 45% left in the first container that we have to work with. Flashbacks continue to come at the same speed as before. The other containers behind are pushing forward. The memories are in queue.

Pedophiles

Pedophiles are generally perceived as perpetrators as there is conceptual confusion, despite both professionals and research showing that not all pedophiles prey on children or that all perpetrators are pedophiles Berlin, (2014); referenced in Nielsen, Askov & Larsen, (2020). It is estimated that 3% to 9% of the general male population feels a sexual attraction to children Wurtele, Simons & Moreno, (2014); referenced in Houtepen, Sijtsema & Bogaerts, (2015). Pedophilia is the only diagnosis in Sweden that lacks a patient association. Seto, 2012; referenced in Houtepen, Sijtsema & Bogaerts, (2015) shows that pedophilia has many similarities with sexual gender orientation such as homosexuality or heterosexuality, it arises early in life, there is a fantasy or desire to engage in romantic behavior and the stability of the sexual preference exists over time. Therefore, Seto suggests that it would be better if pedophilia were considered a sexual orientation, a personal sexuality instead of a disease or a sexual preference that is chosen or in some way learned. The definition of pedophilia is a sexual disorder that, among other things, involves a lasting sexual interest in children. This can manifest itself in fantasies, impulses and in actual sexual abuse of children. According to Miller, (2013); referenced in Blalock & Bourke, (2020), pedophilia only becomes criminal when the individual acts on their urges, fantasies or behavior that violates the boundaries of the law. Therefore, it is important for therapists, the police and other professionals to gain a better understanding and knowledge of pedophilia to prevent pedophiles from going from thought to action. There are currently stable basic assumptions for how we can understand individuals who commit sexual abuse. According to Quinsey, (1986); Seto, (2019); referenced in Pullman, Babchishin & Seto, (2019) there are two broad factors that are present both when initiating and carrying out sexual abuse, atypical sexual interests and antisocial. Atypical sexual interests include sexual interest in prepubertal children (pedophilia) and pubertal children (hebephilia). The antisocial traits include impulsivity, risk-taking, insensitivity and an offensive attitude. Bonta & Andrews (2017) talk about eight different risk factors for perpetrators as the Central Eight, which include an antisocial history, antisocial personality pattern, pro-criminal attitude, pro-criminal associates, substance abuse, deficit of family relationships/marriage and deficit of education/ work and leisure activities. Houtepen, Sijtsema & Bogaerts, (2015) study shows how pedophiles' sexual interest towards children manifests itself. The respondents in the study were pedophiles and they described having fallen in love with a child, that they fantasized about having a romantic relationship with the child. When asked what specifically they found attractive in children, both physical and psychological characteristics were described, their beauty, body shape, behavior such as openness, spontaneity, honesty or naivety.

Individuals with arousal patterns and sexual interests that are considered outside of social norms are often driven into the virtual world where they can act relatively anonymously, without fear of shame or stigmatization. Online forums allow individuals to find others with similar interests, create support groups where they feel validated, and can share sexual scripts Rosenmann & Safir, (2006); referenced in Holt, Blevins & Burkert, (2010). The stigma has been confirmed via Jahnkes et al., (2015); referenced in Nielsen, Aaskov & Larsens, (2020) study where 28% of respondents believed that pedophiles should die regardless of whether they have committed an assault or not and only 5% would consider being friends with a pedophile. Research examining online forums and discussions suggests that pedophiles have a distorted understanding of their interactions with children, often associated with denial and guilt, blaming society for being mistreated, minimizing their own responsibility and the harm to the victim De Young, (1988); Durkin & Bryant, (1999); Nunes & Jung, (2013); O'Halloran & Quayle, (2010); Pogrebin, Poole, & Martinez, (1992).

McAnena et al., (2016) believe that locus of control means that the perpetrator's agency has been externalized, which means that they experience themselves as passive agents in their own lives and that events and consequences are beyond their control or influenced by external factors such as fate, luck or other people with power. Hanson, Gizzarelli, and Scott, (1994); referenced in Blalock & Bourke, (2020) believe that pedophiles often perceive children as motivated and willing participants in sexual activity with adults. Gul et al., (2020) in their qualitative study of incest survivors address several factors that were previously highlighted that try to explain the motives behind incest and the perpetrator's weakened barrier mechanisms via, among other things, Finkelhorn's (1984) theory. He believes that four factors are in a hierarchical relationship to each other and that the perpetrator must; 1) Feeling an emotional exchange with children (emotional congruency), 2) Having a sexual attraction to children (sexual arousal), 3) Feeling inhibited from developing a deep and lasting relationship with an adult partner (blockage), 4) Breaking one's internal blocking mechanism before initiating sexual contacts with children (disinhibition).

Pedophile manual

According to Durkin, (1997); referenced in Blalock & Bourke, (2020) it is well known that sexual offenders use the internet to distribute violent and exploratory files on children. However, what is less well known is the extent to which they share criminal information with like-minded individuals, communication between adults with deviant predictions that aim to validate paraphilia ignition patterns. With the aim of alleviating feelings of guilt and trepidation and to reinforce the belief that sexual contacts with children are harmless or even beneficial. Within the digital networks, pedophiles have the opportunity to spread otherwise unavailable information about techniques and strategies for sexual abuse of children. In their study, Blalock & Bourke (2020) examine pedophile manuals on the internet about information on how to abuse children. A few years ago, *the United States Marshals Service's Behavioral Analysis Unit* (USMS BAU) was tasked with investigating and compiling pedophile manuals online. Investigators from *Internet Crimes Against Children* (ICAC) and over 4500 police officers informed the researchers about how to manuals that circulated online. In order to obtain a manageable final product, a 775-page graphic compilation of pedophile material was created, without visual images of abuse in order not to spread child pornography. The document provides insight into how pedophile networks engage in criminal activity. They seek out like-minded individuals in chat and online forums where they share stories, spread images, videos and provide information that they believe will help them avoid being discovered by the police. The essence is often to help the group of pedophiles to normalize distorted fantasies and minimize unwanted harm that a pedophile experiences from sexual exploitation as a child. Pedophile manuals were analyzed and the texts described strategies and risks associated with abusing children between 2 and 15 years old, within or outside the family. Advice and tips on grooming, how best to find a child and suggestions on how to silence them and avoid being discovered by the police. The study shows confused arguments that the law needs to take into account children's sexual needs, their premise includes a picture that children are sexual beings and if they are not abused, their sexual needs will be unsatisfied. According to Jenkins, (2011); referenced in Holt, Blevins & Burkert, (2010) ethics and political views are often discussed where a social movement for child love is proposed to make their behavior acceptable to the public. Their abuse is often described by them as sex education. Manuals have numerous suggestions on how their exploitation, abuse and even rape can be healthy if carried out correctly (without overt coercion or persuasion). A common theme is that the authors of the manuals use emollient language such as sexual games and child love to rationalize their actions. The manuals describe how to groom the child by suggesting the term sexual play to convince the victim that these are harmless acts or even normative. The manuals are largely designed to reduce the cognitive dissonance that perpetrators may experience. There is a romanticization of abuse that lasts over a long period of time by calling the child his little wife and the abuse is described as a relationship between the perpetrator and the child. In chapters dealing with penetrative training, it becomes clear to the researchers how much physical pain penetrative abuse on a child generates and, according to Blalock & Bourke (2020), it is impossible to escape the realization how harmful it is for the child.

Analyses of pedophile networks and studies of convicted sex offenders show that perpetrators select their victims based on several different factors: access to the child, perceived vulnerability, AoA (Age of attraction) and attraction Lanning, (2010); McAlinden, (2006); Mooney & Ost, (2013); Olson, Daggs, Ellevold, & Rogers, (2007); referenced in Blalock & Bourke, (2020). Since children are available everywhere, the pedophile manuals did not focus on where to find potential victims but on how potential victims become available to the perpetrator. In the long run, it is not about how to get close to a child but how to get close enough to exploit the children, or as it is called kiddie hunting. Perpetrators who groom children can use digital technology to monitor or exercise control over the victims, for example by threatening to spread images or films, so-called sextortion (SOU, 2023). In Holt, Blevin & Burkert

(2010) study, online forums for pedophiles are analyzed where the selection process is described with which children have shown interest through girl moment or boy moment where children in public environments have sought eye contact which pedophiles perceive as a desire to get in touch. The manuals observe that young children are not unsupervised for any length of time, which makes it difficult to get close enough. Here, the perpetrators were advised that if the parents were present, they should not act with excessive interest in the child, as this could arouse suspicion. Many of the manuals specifically described the vulnerability of the children and gave suggestions on how the perpetrator could best exploit the child's immature defense structures. Conte, Wolf & Smith, (1989); referenced in Blalock & Bourke, (2020) found in their study that perpetrators actively tried to identify vulnerable children. The ideal child victim was often quiet and more withdrawn or children who lacked self-confidence and self-esteem. The fear of being discovered is recurrent in the manuals, advice such as traveling far from home, to avoid the possibility of being recognized by family or friends and that the child cannot recognize the perpetrator. According to Kaufman et al., (1998), the manuals often refer to so-called community heroes as a good way to gain access to children. By including themselves in roles such as coaches, school personnel, church personnel and preschool personnel. Here, the children see how the parents interact with the role, which creates trust between the perpetrator and the child. Pedophiles are found where there are children. Based on the pedophile manuals, we gain insight into a dark but structured, well-organized and motivated world. In other countries, it is a matter of course to make pedophiles visible in order to protect children. In the USA, the police post the names, addresses and crimes of pedophiles on a public website, so that everyone knows where the pedophiles live and what they look like. They are not allowed to live more than 300 meters from a place where children can be found. In addition, pedophiles need to report themselves to the police at regular intervals. Pedophile laws have great support throughout the United States, but several human rights organizations claim that pedophile laws are inhumane.

Female perpetrators

Research shows that female perpetrators are often very similar to male perpetrators in terms of background and the way they abuse children (Johnsson & Svedin, 2021).

Harrati, Coulanges, Derivois & Vavassori, (2018); referenced in Johnsson & Svedin, (2021) analyzed 35 judgments regarding the motives of female perpetrators and found four main reasons for committing abuse; a) a sense of power, b) sadism, c) being extremely angry, and d) the pursuit of self-affirmation. According to McCarty (1986), research shows that only 4% of incest perpetrators are mothers. According to Courtois (1988), victims of female perpetrators are younger compared to victims of male perpetrators. The abuse often starts in infancy and continues for 6–11 years and Peter (2009) states that 92% of female perpetrators' victims were 9 years or younger and they discriminated to a lesser extent against boys or girls. They had no clear gender preference. Female perpetrators have a more complex trauma experience compared to male perpetrators (Strickland, 2008). Beckett et al, (2007); Ring, (2005); referenced in Johansson & Svedin, (2021) found that both men and women had an inability to empathize with their victim. Burkey & Benser, (2015); referenced in Johansson & Svedin, (2021) made a comparison between female lone perpetrators of child abuse and those who committed the abuse together with someone else regarding how they rationalized their actions. In both groups, when women were the sole perpetrators and when they committed the abuse together with someone else, excuses were the most common. That the judgment had been impaired due to abuse or a description that it was the child who committed the sexual assault. As in families with generational incest, there was a perception that the abuse was not harmful to the children either physically or psychologically. In the sexual exploitation of children, female perpetrators may be forced to some extent to commit sexual abuse and carry it out reluctantly (Gannon, et al., 2008) or that it is a matter of pure threats and abuse of women to commit sexual abuse of children Matthews et al., (1991); referenced in Johansson & Svedin, (2021).

Elliott, Eldrigde, Ashfield & Beech, (2010); referenced in Haliburn, (2017) argue that knowledge of female perpetrators needs to be acknowledged after information has emerged over the past century. The stereotypical image in society of a perpetrator is narrow and needs to be broadened. Children need to learn that a perpetrator can look anything from your mother, aunt, family friend, sibling or grandfather. The lack of recognition that female perpetrators exist has hindered information gathering, understanding and support for adults, teenagers and children who are victims. Mother-son incest and female pedophilia is still an unexplored and unknown topic. According to Banning, (1989); referenced in Haliburn, (2017) there is still a general reluctance to believe that women are capable of pedophilic acts which is a result of a gender bias. Sexual crimes committed by women are more likely to end up in the hidden, which means that the abuse can continue. Women can engage in more transgressive activities than men in caring for and raising the child without anyone from the outside perceiving it as deviant or strange. For the child, the borderline between acceptable or questionable actions and outright abuse can be particularly confusing. Where did the line go?, when something ordinary has turned into something unpleasant. According to Dahlström-Lannes (1994), boys, unlike girls, do not absolve themselves of guilt when abused by an older female perpetrator, but can instead experience themselves as a skilled seducer who, for example, has seduced an adult woman. The boy frees himself from powerlessness and feelings of guilt by transforming the sexual relationship into an equal one. Mathews and colleagues (1989) developed a typology for female perpetrators with the aim of understanding female perpetrator behavior. They divided the different typologies into; A) Teacher/lover- the woman does not think that the sexual relationship with a child is a harmful relationship, she denies that what is happening is illegal and mainly thinks that it is about love. B) Predisposed- here the woman has her own history of sexual abuse that influences her to commit abuse, mainly on children in her vicinity, who may be her own. There is no man behind the abuse. C) Forced by a man- here the woman does not commit sexual abuse without a man's presence and their victim is usually their own or a common child. Less common categories are; D) Experimenting and exploiting, which is a woman who is often younger and who exposes younger boys. Can probably be someone who is babysitting. E) Mentally ill- women who exhibit psychotic characteristics but do not need to be diagnosed.

The model has been developed by several researchers and has served as a starting point in the work of exploring new typologies. Ahlmonde et al., (2017) found three themes in addition to the already described typologies as A) *Involvement*- the dominant theme is that the woman tries to develop a pseudo-intimate consensual relationship with the child by, for example, buying gifts or giving the child alcohol, but also by, for example, blackmail. B) *Control*- the second most common theme where the perpetrator takes control of the child mentally and physically, C) *Hostility*- the least common theme where threats, violence and coercion were used. In the Norwegian article *No penis, no harm when women commit assault* The authors write about the serious consequences of sexual abuse of a child. The article focuses primarily on the psychological damage, but also addresses physical damage. Women harm children to a lesser extent during sexual abuse than men do physically, but when it does happen, the damage to the victim is more serious. The damage is aggravated if the female perpetrator has been under the influence of drugs or alcohol. Younger children were found to be more physically injured than older children (Nystad, Haugland, Nygaard, Solvik, Vik and Lindström, 2011).

Attachment theory considers the bond between a mother and child to be crucial and the basis for the child to develop healthy relationships with other people later in life (Bowlby, 1988). When the perpetrator is a mother, Cannon & Cortoni, (2010); referenced in Haliburn, (2017) argue that this entails further aggravating circumstances of separation from the mother, an increased need for closeness and validation of the child's existence in a symbiotic dance, which can lead to psychosis. Margolis, (1977); referenced in Haliburn, (2017) describes that unlike girls who are exposed to incest by their mother, boys can experience a feeling of feeling special or *exceptional* with grandiose fantasies of being *king of the world.* My experience of patients with the mother as the perpetrator is that it is more seductive in its character where the mother often projects agency onto the child, especially the son. Since boys have a more visible sexually involuntary response via erection, shame and guilt feelings can be particularly tangible and an experience of having participated in the sexual violence. The abuse of mothers has often begun in a nursing moment such as genital stimulation when showering, changing diapers, or cleaning body openings which then turned into sexual abuse which often creates confusion in the dividing line when closeness becomes abuse. Here, as a therapist, you need to go through the abuse and clearly clarify which moments are questionable or inappropriate in the transitional phase and then obvious abuse. For all nursing situations, abuse situations were not abuse situations. Ogden (1989) believes that this very experience that abuse can progress from a care situation to abuse can make the victim experience the start of the abuse as benign and can have positive feelings that later have a negative psychological impact with effects such as developing an addiction, sexual problems as an adult and self-harming behavior. The boy's psychological development is hindered by hypersexual behavior from the mother. Old Freudian concepts such as becoming castrated by their mother become useful in understanding. As a female psychotherapist to a victim of incest with a mother as the perpetrator, the transference can be challenging. One of the psychotherapists in Haliburn's study (2017) describes that she felt like a dirty mother and that she almost hated the patient in the countertransference and needed, like Winnicott's (1949) theory, to return the projection in a melted form. The transference in the therapy room can sometimes feel overwhelming and limitless, the child's early attachment trauma moves in all parts of the material and is projected mercilessly, making it difficult to distinguish between what is the therapist's and what is the patient's feelings. It is even more difficult for a victim to understand the motive behind the abuse when the perpetrator is the mother. She must really have hated me. It is a common feeling for girls and I was chosen for boys.

Misogynistic attitudes

When it comes to sexual violence against women in general, psychologist Johanna Läth (DN 2025) at the Swedish Prison and Probation Service addresses four risk factors found in men who rape. According to the Swedish Council for Crime Prevention, the victim is a woman or girl in 92% of all reported rapes in Sweden, and in almost all cases the perpetrator is a man. Misogynistic attitudes where the perpetrator believes he has the right to have sex with women regardless of how it turns out for the woman or derogatory attitudes are considered criminal. A second factor concerns the ability to self-regulate impulsivity or that the perpetrator is angry at the time of the rape. The third risk factor shows that perpetrators generally tend to have difficulties with relationships, often with elements of jealousy and conflicts. The fourth risk factor relates to the sexuality of the perpetrator, which may involve paraphilias. Rape often involves physical violence, which is an important means of carrying out the assaults, purely instrumentally. But it can also be about the violence fulfilling a function, linked to power and control which is what the perpetrator wants. The violence can represent sadistic traits in the perpetrator that they enjoy or get excited by seeing someone else suffer which then increases the sexual charge in the perpetrator. It is almost exclusively men who abuse children and women and a significant majority of the victims are girls and women. According to Larsson. et al., (2002); referenced in Kaliray & Drife, (2004) it is 2–5 times more common for girls to be subjected to sexual abuse and in their study from (2002) 98% of the perpetrators were men. It is not all men, but (almost) only men. According to Anders Ahlqvist, IT crime specialist at the Police, the fact that it is a male perpetrator is the only common denominator. Child pornography consumers are not necessarily the stereotypical loner, but there are men of all ages and professions, according to a survey conducted by Netclean, which 400 police officers in different countries were asked to answer. In 40% of cases, the perpetrator lived with a partner and/or with children nearby. Research on porn addiction suggests that men who have excessive porn consumption become tolerant and need to move on to rougher material to experience the same satisfaction, and that the roughest of all material is child rape. However, it is a myth that only women suffer from sexual trauma and that men are both culturally and biologically influenced to minimize or deny the trauma they have been exposed to. There is a lot of research that describes typologies of male perpetrators and how they rationalize, theorize and cognitively explain the crimes they commit. In Wards, (2000); referenced in Johansson & Svedin, (2021), study reveals a difference regarding explanatory models between women and men, namely that female perpetrators considered it a right to abuse children. Regarding men's explanatory models, it was described 1) *What is harmful? There* is a general perception among perpetrators that sexual activities between adults and children are not necessarily harmful. Women did not experience harming children in the same way as men, which led them to see themselves as saviors by participating in the abuse and not leaving the children alone with the male perpetrator. 2) *Children as sexual beings,* a perception that children as adults are sexual beings motivated by desire which includes sexual desire. One difference between female and male perpetrators in the study was that women believed that it was more specific children and not children in general who were sexual beings. Which may later explain boys' experience of having *been selected and special* by the mother. 3) *Uncontrollable,* a perception that the acts of abuse are externally controlled and could not be sheltered. 4) *Right,* a perception that the man is all-powerful and therefore must also have his sexual needs satisfied.

Treatment SAIS, 5-6 CPTSD and DID

Talking through

Suzette Boon coined the term talking through. The method involves talking to all parts within the patient at the same time. Since shifts take energy and it is time-consuming to talk to one part at a time, the most effective way to talk to all parts is through talking through (Putnam, 1989; referenced in Howell, 2011). If all parts can listen now, I would like to introduce myself to you as a therapist. You start by giving all parts that want permission to listen. When all parts are listening, you can address the part you want to talk to. You can provide psychoeducation by telling them that you were raised by people who hurt you and wanted you to obey, but they are no longer present. You no longer have to follow their rules. Different parts will have different ease in building a working alliance with the therapist throughout the course of therapy. Conflicts between different parts that may think it is dangerous, I must never trust anyone, she seems to genuinely care about me and understands me, this kind lady can take care of me, maybe she can be my mother, I have to do exactly as she says to get what I want or she is after something, people just want to take advantage of us. By talking through, you as a therapist come into contact with parts that may be shy, do not usually come forward or that lie more below the surface. The therapist needs to gain knowledge about which part is afraid of a working alliance in order to be able to approach all parts. When in the initial part you examine the patient's inner structure, the intervention of talking through is a valuable tool. For a patient who is not fragmented, a talking through intervention seems incomprehensible; what would it be like if I spoke to all your parts?, they do not understand what the therapist means. For a person with DID, it is often the first time they are seen, that someone understands them, speaks directly to them. For the DID patient, it is obvious that they are divided into different participants, they do not know anything else. Many times they believe that everyone else is also divided. The first time someone talks through is usually a milestone in therapy for patients with DID and an important key to making the correct diagnosis.

The Trauma curve by Dr. Eric Wolterstroff

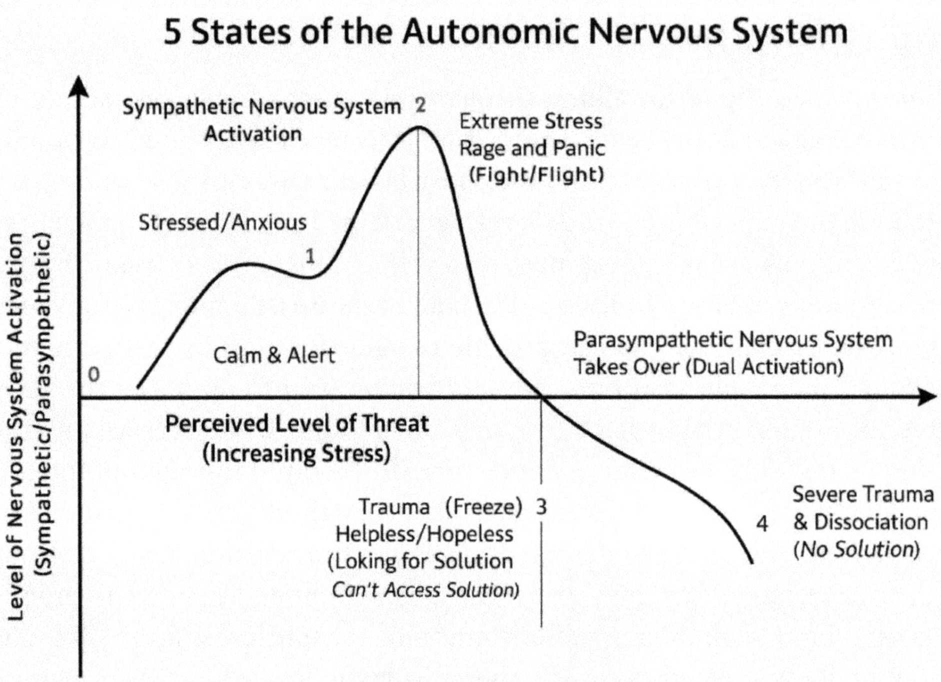

Stage 0: Calm, regulated, alert
Stage 1: Low stress, tension, irritability, uncomfortable
Stage 2: High stress, panic, anger, fight/flight
Stage 3: Double condition, anxiety plus collapse, exhaustion
Stage 4: Disconnection, numb, no emotions, dissociation

What can be called the map of the nervous system has been developed by Eric Wolterstorff, Ph.D., based onPeter Levin's work to observe and understand the nervous system's response to rest and stress, in his dissertation *Accumulated Stress, Reserve Capacity and Disease* (1976). The model in its entirety can be found in Levin's student Eric Wolterstoff's book *Love and Trauma* (2011). Wolterstorff refined Levin's method by combining meditative awareness of the nervous system. He discovered that certain defense structures could be completed and strengthened through conscious focus and repetition. He also took elements from memory science such as distinguishing between semantic (the part of long-term memory that stores general knowledge, facts, and concepts), procedural (the ability to perform and remember skills and procedures), and episodic (the ability to remember certain personal events and experiences that have occurred) memory. The trauma curve is a powerful tool that clinicians can use in the treatment of traumatized patients.

Peter Levine initially used a model in which he describes how a gazelle is chased on the savanna by a lion. He meant that in stage 0. The gazelle lies down and rests after eating, she is at rest, and has a calm nervous system. In stage 1. The gazelle sees a lion further away and experiences mild stress, becomes uncomfortable and the system begins to prepare for stage 2. Now the lion has seen the gazelle and runs with full force towards its prey. The gazelle tries to escape the lion and runs for its life across the savanna, is in high stress, panic and in full fight/flight mode. In stage 3. The lion has caught up with the gazelle and has taken a big bite to the neck of the gazelle which is playing dead, is in collapse and completely exhausted, but there is still some hope that the lion can let go and the gazelle can escape. In stage 4, all hope is gone, the pride of lions has arrived and everyone is eating the gazelle, which is stunned by neurotransmitters and endorphins that are released to counteract the pain, and the gazelle is in dissociation.

When using the model to describe the stages of a rape, it can be clarified where in the trauma curve the patient is during different parts of the assault. In stage 0. the child is lying down and resting, in stage 1. She hears someone walking up the stairs, the door opens and the perpetrator comes and starts touching the child, she experiences mild stress, her body becomes tense and uncomfortable. In stage 2. The rape is in its most intense stage, here any penetration occurs and the pain is at its highest for the child who experiences the fight/flight response, anger and panic. The pain, abandonment and understanding that the child will not escape lead to the activation of the parasympathetic nervous system (PNS is a part of the autonomic nervous system that is active during rest and recovery that acts as a counterforce to the sympathetic nervous system fight/flight). In stage 3. The child is completely in the abuser's power, stunned, in collapse and dissociating because in stage 4. The child has completely left his own body and finds himself in a situation without a solution.

There are many different ways to work with breaking dissociation. In my experience, the most important thing is to know that it exists, to be able to map it via the trauma curve and to be able to provide psychoeducation. Eric Wolterstoff's curve is an effective and educational tool for both mapping and psychoeducation. Patients often recognize themselves, and it can be extremely helpful for patients to be able to be reminded that; Yes, everything feels hopeless right now, and that's because you are in stage three (not because it is and will always be hopeless). Or: Yes, it feels like you are completely disconnected and alone and as if you have no body, because right now you are in stage four (not because you do not feel and will never feel contact with your body or with any other person).

Eric Wolterstoff's book Love and Trauma provides a very good basis for how to work systematically with the dissociation curve, and break the dissociation. He calls the method containment and exposure therapy. Saj Razvi, one of Eric Wolterstoff's former students, has developed the method further by adding psychedelics to the same process, and calls it Psychedelic Somatic Inter Relational Psychotherapy. When you work with containment and selective inhibition (meaning that you inhibit or block a specific reaction or process) you do not avoid the dissociation, but you work with it. It is a new way of looking at dissociation and tolerance windows, and training in the method can be transformative and challenging, but is highly recommended.

Top of mind model SAIS 5-6

Many therapists feel great uncertainty when they encounter a fragmented system in the therapy room. Several of my patients testify to treatments that have either been terminated or that they have been forwarded on to another therapist when they have switched and shown other parts of themselves in the therapy process. However, many clinicians appreciate working with the image of multiple parts within the patient's mind and the dissociative structure can be used as an explanatory model. From this perspective, none of us is a "singular" unit but a well-developed organized aggregation (a method that involves combining and summarizing data) of self-parts that are integrated within us to varying degrees. In this way, working with DID patients "multiples" can lead to new ways of providing good psychotherapy to people who do not have multiple personalities (Howell, 2011). There are several different ways to address dissociative parts within the patient. You can ask to speak to a part directly, *talking through or* ask the host if it can ask for a certain part inside. There is great value in talking to individual parts directly to find out how they are feeling, what their role in the system is, what they have been through and what they need. We need to explain to each individual part that they have an important role in the system, they have arisen for a reason and they have an important part in helping the system to heal. The vast majority of parts come up naturally in therapy or in different memory paths when they have something to tell. It is usually not difficult to get different dissociative parts to go back into the system when the session is over. Usually they help each other as a cooperative and understand that the session must end at a certain time and the patient must switch to an adult part before they leave the therapy room as it is not safe for a 4 year old to cross the street or take the bus home by themselves. If a younger part does not want to go back into the system, you can reassure the part that we will see each other again soon.

For a DID patient, it makes a big difference if the therapist can recognize shifts and work with the part of the self in the therapy room. For example, if a patient does not recognize or remember what we talked about in the previous session, in traditional psychotherapy it can be interpreted as resistance or anxiety, but it can also be due to dissociation and that another part was in the therapy room the previous session. Trauma is complex and the therapist needs to have solid experience, be trained in different methods to be able to treat traumatic memories and have established a working alliance before the work of getting to know and mapping the different parts begins. As a trauma therapist, you need to be well acquainted with traumatic transference and countertransference and have the ability to handle strong emotions in the therapy room. I recommend Lifespan Integration as a trauma treatment method for sexually abused patients in SAIS 1-4 but not for SAIS 5-6, here psychodynamic three-phase therapy and free associations need to be the basis of the treatment together with Allison Miller's method of how to treat trauma memories. I have developed a method where clinicians and therapists with different experiences of dissociation and DID can gain the courage to begin to investigate and continue their learning in the unique world of dissociation. I usually describe the unconscious and classical psychodynamic psychotherapy as an infinitely large puzzle. When the patient enters the therapy room, neither the therapist nor the patient knows how the patient's puzzle will be created and developed. Each new part of the material that the patient presents becomes a new puzzle piece and together we put together the patient's life puzzle through the treatment, which includes memories, feelings, thoughts and pieces from the conscious and unconscious. My work as a therapist is to see connections, make interventions, ask questions and interpret the puzzle that emerges. When the patient is fragmented, each part within the patient has its own puzzle that needs to be put together. Each part has its own memories, feelings, experiences, characteristics and material. As usual, the patient's traumatic memories are treated in an age-appropriate manner (based on the part's perceived age) and with free associations as a basis. In a fragmented patient, no part of the life puzzle resembles the other. When we integrate parts with the host part later in the therapy process, we simply put the pieces of the puzzle together. By the host part becoming aware of what another part has been through when we have taken down the dissociative barriers, they are joined at the edges and grow into a larger common puzzle. A picture that becomes clear to the patient about what integration means, no parts disappear, they are only treated so as not to arouse triggers or flashbacks and are then joined with the host part. With sometimes 100s of parts within the patient, the puzzle can become infinitely large. But therapeutically, it is just the same process that is repeated. I have developed the Top of mind model from an eclectic perspective where different ways of stabilizing, providing psychoeducation, exposing and treating trauma are used in a patient-focused way to treat CPTSD and DID. Different therapeutic principles have been developed to make all parts feel safe in the room and dare to come forward, which is required when facing such a complex system as a DID patient. Not all DID patients will be able to go through all three phases, but even if they do not progress to the next phase, the model leads to increased functionality, well-being and increased quality of life for the patient. In MDMA-assisted therapy, it is said that the participant needs to trust her *inner healing intelligence*. The patient is the expert and we teach the patient to trust themselves which leads to them regaining a sense of agency and a certain sense of power. The therapist's responsibility is to create a non-judgmental environment that psychologically offers the patient to speak openly and honestly. This requires the therapist to listen to the subtext beyond the spoken word to reach a deeper meaning about the patient. By acknowledging the other's suffering and validating the patient's feelings and being genuinely sincere, the empathetic approach creates a reduction in feelings of abandonment in the patient. Empathetic listening means that you as a therapist may need to admit that you do not have all the answers. According to the Multidisciplinary Association for Psychedelic Studies (MAPS), the following points are important components of active and empathetic listening.

Minimal encouragement, verbal or non-verbal
Invitations instead of directions
Paraphrasing, to refer when speaking in someone else's words
Reflect
Validation
Insure and wait in
Allow the patient to come to their own conclusions

By addressing the patient's own ability to heal and grow, we are talking about the body's own healing ability. If a patient goes to the doctor with a wound, the doctor will wash the wound, remove any obstacles to healing, and may create favorable conditions for healing, but it is the body that heals the wound. In the same way, the psyche has an internal healing ability to heal.

Top of mind- The model is divided into:

An initial stabilization and mapping phase of previously known parts
A trauma treatment phase where memory pathways are followed according to the Top of mind model
An integrative phase with explanatory models is developed as well as psychoeducation

Phase 1: Initial stabilization and mapping

To undertake the arduous work of treating CPTSD and DID patients in SAIS grade 4-6, we as therapists need to enter with a *Beginner's mind.* We need to have an open approach and accept that we do not understand. It will take a long time before we get a first grasp of the therapy process and we need to continue working even when we have doubts. Remember that without doubt you are not wise. Kluft (1993); referenced in Howell, (2011) believes that the pace and intensity need to be in tune with the patient's current vulnerability and resilience, "the slower you work the faster you get there". It is therefore not a model with a rigid time frame. We always need to remember that patients with CPTSD and DID have created a dissociative structure for good reasons. A large part of the therapy will be about the patient grieving their childhood. In the first phase of therapy, it is of great importance to stabilize the patient so that all parts feel safe and so that the therapist can map out what the patient's inner family or system looks like. The patient will initially experience a destabilization, but this is often short-lived. Here, the therapist needs to work on establishing a sense of security, safety and openness. But also work on ensuring that the patient has a more stable existence through interventions regarding self-care, day and night, routines, safety, food, social support systems, health, work, rest and play. People with CPTSD and DID often have difficulty with trust, which is why the working alliance and the patient's skills and resources will be tested when treatment starts. Any therapy that involves revisiting the trauma time in order to treat traumatic memories will temporarily increase anxiety and activation and awaken other strong emotions within the patient. Therefore, in this first phase we need to work with skill exercises that strengthen the patient, as well as sensorimotor and somatic psychotherapeutic techniques to understand psychological symptoms based on psychological states through psychoeducation. We also need to spend time explaining the therapy process and talking about the patient's expectations, while explaining that they will sometimes experience strong overwhelming emotions and they will feel strong feelings towards the therapist. Psychoeducation should also include general knowledge about trauma and dissociation. Here, Suzette Boon's book of exercises can help to deal with trauma-related dissociation. Psychoeducation initially contributes to creating a sustainable working alliance but is useful throughout the therapy process. Patients with trauma can sometimes react with extreme reactions to something the therapist has said or done or not said or done. Other aspects of psychoeducation include breathing exercises, exercises on how to calm the body, foundational techniques and methods for being able to calm oneself. For example, teaching the patient to breathe in through the nose and out through the mouth. A crucial part of the initial phase is to get to know all the parts known so far and teach them to improve the internal communication between them. There is a gain in getting to know them one by one or as Kluft (2000); referenced in Howell, (2011) believes that it is neither necessary nor recommended to bring all parts together into a common consciousness too early in therapy. In the initial part of therapy, we should encourage the host part to listen inwardly and to ask inwardly. We help the parts to become more aware of each other's existence and to come forward. They need to learn to help each other, listen to each other and jointly break down dissociative barriers in the system. We break the barriers by uncovering dissociated material and by following memory paths and gaining access to details in trauma memories and processing them. When the patient listens inwardly, they get images, words or flowing thoughts. Many times the patient hears several different voices/parts within themselves that want to say their thing, sometimes they have contradictory opinions and we have to negotiate together. Do you want to think out loud? is one of my most common interventions. Here we bring out the patient's inner dialogue in the therapy room and can think together.

As therapists, we also need to believe in and convey the patient's inner ability and capacity to heal their traumas. Before trauma treatment, we need to convey hope, that we have seen the end of the movie, you are sitting here. Everything we are going to go through is already within you, it has already happened. How we describe their symptoms needs to be linked to their traumatic experiences, not primarily their diagnoses. The patient gets flashbacks because it is the brain's way of communicating that she needs to remember in order to heal her traumas and injuries. Once upon a time, you forgot, but now you remember. It happened then but feels like the present because the memory is so strong. Miller (2014) describes flashbacks as our mind regurgitating memories. Different patients name their inner world in different ways, here we need to find a common term for the patient's inner system together so that all parts can recognize each other. Sometimes it is important for the patient that we address them as a we instead of a I. Through an initial mapping of the patient's inner world, we learn which parts are prominent in the therapy room and when the patient changes. Mapping means that all parts that the patient is aware of so far are written down, named if possible, age, gender, sexual affiliation, sexual orientation, voice position, special tics, what trauma they are connected to, who is its perpetrator, which parts the part is connected to or is otherwise aware of. Some parts may have special characteristics such as being allergic to something, having pain in some part of the body, being right or left handed, having a disability, having different blood pressure, speaking different languages, being playful, mischievous, angry, afraid, talented, only doing as they are told, etc. Here it is valuable to ask the patient to physically create an image of their inner world, that different images or objects may symbolize different parts of the patient. One patient crocheted different flowers that represented different parts. By mapping the inner world, we as therapists gain information about how many parts are active so far and how they are connected to each other. More parts will emerge through the therapy process. But above all, we need to tell the patient that when you hear your inner parts, they are only communicating with you and they need you to communicate back to them. They were the ones who made you survive your childhood when your life was in danger both physically and mentally, so they need to be treated with respect, care and gratitude. You cannot get rid of them, but if they become connected to the rest of you, by sharing your memories, they will change (Miller, 2014). The mapping also needs to include information about previous therapy experience, therapists, what they have talked about in previous therapies, why they ended, who ended the therapy, any conflicts with the therapist, attachment issues and expectations. An important part to map is the patient's native language, some parts may only understand a certain language. Other parts just want to write and cannot speak. Before the therapy moves on to the next step, the therapist needs to have an insight into how severe the dissociative symptoms are, how the patient organizes their self, who is the host part?, other comorbid symptoms such as addiction, self-harm, anorexia, internal resources, support system, family, social/financial situation.

During the mapping, we get an entry point to begin to understand the patient's internal system and we learn where the major areas or time spans of trauma are found. We also learn who knows each other, who is the host part, who comes to therapy. It is equally important to map the parts that do not want to come to the therapy room, those that show resistance or do not dare to build a relationship of attachment, we accept that there are parts with resistance and parts that actively oppose the therapy process. By working with the patient's resources and skills and abilities, we learn how their possibilities to mentalize are structured, whether they have any safe points, places or parts within themselves. If the patient does not have a safe place within themselves, we need to work on creating one. We also need to map what triggers/activates and calms the patient in the form of places, smells, relationships, people, sounds, etc. Since DID patients vary in the number of parts from 2 to in the thousands, the mapping needs to take into account that not all parts will appear. When the patient has several hundred parts, the parts are usually divided into groups such as the mother parts, the child parts, the adult parts, the teenage parts, the perpetrator parts, etc. Through the mapping, we activate several memory pathways within the patient, initiating several neural processes without going into depth in specific memories. This means that we activate the patient without them becoming overwhelming. Most DID patients find the mapping exciting and many child parts are excited that someone is showing interest. Some want to talk and have a lot to tell, while others may be mute or want someone else to speak for them. They often find it an exciting but also frightening process to get to know each other. It often arouses surprise in the patient about how many parts there are when you put them together. But sometimes the mapping can be met with resistance as the perpetrators often used different names to call their victims in order to give them a punishment, a certain task or an assignment. The patient can sometimes name their inner parts without any problem, but may not want to. Talking to someone outside can also be associated with serious threats about what would happen to them if they tell, which we need to keep with us throughout the therapy process. The importance of giving the right intervention to the right part is crucial in therapy. Once you talk to the right part, a simple intervention or psychoeducation can lead to major changes. The mapping should be entered into the medical record system so that during the course of therapy you can see if parts are added or if they are integrated and become fewer in number.

Different DID patients describe their internal systems with different models. One patient describes a planetary system, with stars and galaxies. The more activated the parts are, the closer they are to the Earth, the more disoriented the patient feels, the further away from the Earth the part she is in is. When she doesn't want to think about anything, wants to switch or wants to disconnect and dissociate, she moves traumatic memory paths and parts further out into the galaxy to function for the day. In therapy, we work with the planetary system as a resource when treating the patient's trauma. After we have gone through a traumatic memory, the part that has been treated is allowed to move far out into the planetary system to rest. No perpetrators can reach her there, it is too far away. Another patient has built a fantasy castle by the sea, Villa vila, where God protects and all the children live separately and the adult parts separately. We have created rooms where I, as a therapist, can enter. We often start the session with all the child parts and I sitting together on the leaves of a sunflower mat to go over who needs to talk today. As a therapist, I often have a child on my lap, someone finds what we are talking about tiring and walks away, and they learn to take care of and comfort each other. The adult parts live in the house next door and take care of cooking and other household chores that the child cannot handle or finds boring.

Others create spaces on their property where the children can feel safe and play after they have told what they have been through. For the vast majority of children, it is enough to just tell what they have been through, to someone they feel safe with. They also often want the host to listen in to get to know them. Once they have told their story, they become like normal children and want to do what non-traumatized children do, play, paint and fool around.

Some children are naughty, others are ill-mannered, some want to play with me as a therapist. With a patient, we always start the session by playing rock, scissors and bag with the children. The child parts that have been released from trauma often gain a great deal of trust in the therapist and you need to treat the relationship with them carefully. Other DID systems are more disorganized, a patient likens their inner system to a dysfunctional school class without a teacher. The patients' inner systems embroider themselves through the treatment and I often ask them to write down their worlds and then put them in the journal to be able to follow the development.

In the encounter with child parts, it is easy for one's therapeutic principles and boundaries to be displaced. How can you say no to a child who is afraid, living in a time of trauma and just wants us to send a voice message? Even though we have agreed that all contact must go through the adult parts. Shusta-Hochberg, (2004); referenced in Howell, (2011) notes that it is important to remember that the patient is an adult, the child parts are just ego-state-like personalities and not real children. Some child parts may mature and grow up during the course of therapy and other child parts remain the same age throughout therapy. Different parts may have different relationships with their perpetrators. Some may speak of their father idealized, as a warm, caring person and some may hate him. Many times the patient may have parts that are referred to as twins such as the good twin and the evil twin. In the therapy room, all parts need to know that we are here with you, as a therapist I need to make sure that all parts feel safe enough for the work that we are going to do during the session. We have to remember that the patient may have spent the last two or three decades trying to pretend that certain parts do not exist, ignoring them, so it is not surprising that they do not trust you or consult the patient's adult parts. Learning to speak to their inner parts means that the patient thinks the question inside and then sees what words or thoughts come to them, they are often surprised. Sometimes a part leaks a strong feeling inside to the host part. When waves of memory pathways emerge and take over the body, we need to encourage the patient to let the waves wash through them, allow involuntary movements to run out and to trust their feelings. Here we may need to help the patient not to work against the wave but to follow it. As therapists, we need to constantly be aware of how old the patient is in different memory paths, stay with them when they feel like someone is going to hurt them. Ask humble questions, I wonder? so that all parts dare to emerge. The patient will feel ambivalent about sharing certain parts of themselves with the therapist as there are parts that protect the system. Your past does not exist now, how can we rewrite it together and what do you want me to do now? When we go through the trauma, it passes. The patient needs the therapist's support in the process to understand different parts of themselves. When memories are uncovered, it is not about being a detective but about what the memories mean to the patient. We need to support the process even if we do not understand it. Patients with CPTSD and DID are empathetic and intuitive and therefore we as therapists need to be authentic and speak the truth.

Phase 2 The trauma treatment

In the second phase, we as therapists need to allow the inner healing process to progress instead of avoiding traumatic memories. We need to remind the patient that even though it is terribly painful to bring up memories from the traumatic time, they cannot hurt you anymore, they are just memories. At the same time, we respect the patient's resistance to entering the treatment phase, which manifests itself in different ways based on the patient's SAIS degree. In SAIS 1-2, the patient will show traditional therapeutic resistance, in SAIS degree 3-4, the patient's psychological defenses will be activated, and in SAIS degree 5-6, the protective ego will emerge.

A SAIS 6 patient with DID describes their brain as a bunch of tabs in an operating system on a computer, they are full of sounds, short videos, still images, moments and behind each tab there are 100 more tabs. A complexity that the therapist needs to take into account is the division that the patient has within themselves that has arisen for good reasons to protect the individual, a built-in resilience that allows them to switch in unbearable situations. It becomes dual as the fragmentation counteracts the effectiveness of the psychotherapeutic trauma treatment. When the therapist is about to approach the trauma, the patient switches in the room. The defense is activated during the treatment. Many times it is a child part that is active in the room when the patient receives trauma treatment, as it is the part that was created during the trauma, is the carrier of the trauma or was the one who experienced the abuse. As a therapist, you need to relate to the age of the patient/child part in an age-appropriate manner. Sometimes the material may feel inappropriate to talk about with a child of the child part's age, but it was also not appropriate when the memory was encoded into the hands of the perpetrator. But it is important to remember that they are not ordinary children, they are child parts that have been given the job of holding information or emotions that have been too overwhelming for the host part to handle, sometimes children can handle things that adults cannot (Miller, 2014).

Uncovering memories via memory pathways is based on Freud's theory of free association. That the patient is allowed to associate freely to reach the material in the unconscious. A psychoanalytic technique where the patient can freely and without censorship express all thoughts, memories and feelings that appear in the conscious in order to gain access to the unconscious. By moving forward in memory pathways via free associations, we ensure that the patient does not become overwhelmed, "flooded" or stuck in memory. The unconscious is probably Freud's most fundamental concept in psychoanalysis and psychodynamic psychotherapy. The concept became something that ordinary people could understand and think about, not just philosophers. The concept shows that our actions, thoughts, what motivates us are more complex and have a tendency to expand and spread. How the trauma treatment phase is designed depends on which theoretical method the therapist is working with. In order to regulate the intensity within the memory pathways, it is good to use "muting" techniques. Together with the patient, we visualize that they have a remote control that they can use to rewind and forward in their memory. They can press pause, raise or lower the sound or slow down the speed of the scene, they can remove the light in the image or make all the images smaller or as if they are looking at them from a distance, but above all they can turn it off. Allison Miller also talks about putting all the emotions, other scenes, sounds, images, pain, etc. in a container with a tap at the bottom. You fill the container with memory fragments and then let the container slowly empty the material so that the patient does not become overwhelmed. The tap lets the water/memories flow through the container in a calm current. The patient can choose to rewind the memory path, the therapist guides by asking what happens next? and the patient tells us where we are going. Seeing the memory as a scene can be an asset when the memory is too painful to bear its full intensity. It helps the patient to gain some form of control. Incomplete memories and feelings that one has begun to work with can, according to (Kluft, 1989; referenced in Howell, 2011), be locked in a vault with the therapist to be retrieved and unlocked at the next opportunity or as he calls it, to leak slowly. However, there are difficulties with the model of completely locking the material in until the next opportunity as trauma memories have a tendency to leak through the system to the host part. The patient needs to be prepared to deal with certain memories in the memory path, details or fragments via flashbacks on their own between sessions. There is simply too much material in a DID patient to take all the memories during the sessions, but not all the details need to be available or revealed to the patient for the memory to be integrated into the system.

According to Howell, 2011, a conflict forms within the patient's system that is only found when working with multiple personalities. When one part has shared a painful memory that affects more parts within the patient, a conflict arises. The parts that carry the painful feelings connected to the memory become desperate to share their pain with the therapist. But then, I also want to tell you now. Other parts may be just as desperate to keep memories secret. This conflict looks different when working with memory paths, as the patient has the opportunity to switch between different parts and bring up different fragments of memories based on what is first, top of mind. The patient's system determines which part of the memory is to be treated and which part is to be active. By asking what happens next? The patient himself moves on to the part that is next in line and wants to speak. The parts soon learn the system and that they have to queue up to be allowed to speak. In my experience, the parts become more frustrated and the conflict more visible when the therapist stops at a memory to go through it from beginning to end, when the memory is not encoded into a narrative structure with a certain given time order. There is a protective effect of following the patient's memory paths and how the memories are encoded and how they are connected to each other. A part may have been active during many abuses and then that part carries fragments of several different abuses at different ages.

My experience has taught me to follow the patient's system, we are guided through different memory paths based on the patient's inherent ability to self-heal. Trauma memories are often connected to each other in memory paths just as positive memories are connected to each other in memory paths. In a DID system, memories are often connected like in a queue system. When a memory is processed, other traumatic memories are activated, which are in a queue or are in tabs behind the memory that triggered the memory path. You often only have time to get a little bit into the memory path during the trauma treatment session. Therefore, the treatment often continues when the patient goes home and has left the therapy room via flashbacks that can be very tiring for the patient. Here, the therapist needs to be available to the patient and more sessions may need to be carried out within the next few days. The problem is that neither the patient nor the therapist knows how activating different memory paths are before the work begins. In the initial phase, the patient needs to be taught to lock parts of the memory in a box with a lid or in a box and that they can only look a little under the lid to see what is inside. This can give an indication of what we are getting into. If the memory cannot be locked in a box, the patient can be asked to look at the memory from afar. It usually does not take long to look at a memory (a few seconds), but then the therapist can get an indication of how activating the memory in the memory path is. When a memory path with a string of different traumatic events has been processed, the patient often temporarily becomes calm, tired and experiences symptom relief. In the mapping in the initial phase, an estimate is made of how many trauma memories may be present within the patient's system. For DID patients, this can involve over 1000 traumatic memories of torture-like abuse. It is not possible to go through all the memories in the therapy room, but the treatment needs to be designed so that the patient can do some of the work on their own at home. The contact that takes place between sessions where the patient writes down memories, paints, records memories, talks to AI or with relatives is an important part of the treatment. For each memory path that is treated, the patient will feel safer for the next memory path as they learn where in the trauma curve they are. They learn the process and that when they go through it, it will end. There is always a quiet period before the next memory path is treated, as if the body is resting for the next healing phase. There are several different trauma methods that govern which memories should be treated, in what order and when in the process. Working with DID patients requires that you adapt your previous training and orientations to the patient sitting in front of you, the method can never be adapted to the patient. One of the challenges in working with DID patients is that you need to be willing to work with exactly what comes up. Bring courage into the patient to dare to face the material, remind them that nothing will come up that is not already there. Whatever comes up is something that the patient is already carrying around without being aware of it. For patients in SAIS grade 4-6 with CPTSD and DID, we should control as little as possible but primarily follow the patient's own ability and capacity. By working with*Top of mind*, what is first, at the forefront, at the moment gives the most flashbacks, what the patient herself wants to work on, most activating in the present, we let the system choose the direction itself and we follow how the memories are connected to each other. This does not mean that we let the patient take care of themselves but that they are allowed to be involved in controlling their own treatment. The Top of Mind model also means that it is the patient who chooses the strength or intensity of the session. Sometimes the patient needs to rest in therapy and the Top of Mind is then some topic for the day that is not activating. Different memories are connected via different memory paths that activate each other. Traumatic memories are interconnected, when we treat a memory it will automatically activate other memories that are in the same path or associate with each other. Only the patient knows what this association looks like, which means that the process is difficult for the therapist to control or feel in control of. For each child part we retrieve from the trauma time, we need to remind them that they will never be in this situation again, it is completely over. What is uncovered is uncovered forever. Afterwards, the memory takes on a different quality, the patient remembers it as dull or in a different color, it is now just part of the total puzzle. It becomes something terrible that happened to them a long time ago but does not exist in the present. Through treatment, the nature of the memory gradually changes and the patient gradually improves by alleviating the symptoms of PTSD. There are parts within the patient that actively work to weaken the working alliance, never build it up or destroy it. Perpetrator parts that need to be met with love and respect but that manipulate and rule. New parts require new parts of you as a therapist. We can doubt ourselves as therapists but love yourself as a person (MAPS, 2015). Some parts need a clearer framework while other parts need a non-directive therapist who is more restrictive with interventions. The timing of when the therapist chooses to say something is crucial, so that the right part gets the right information. The more material we probe through interventions, the less information we get about where the patient is. By holding back connections, letting the parts get to know each other at their own pace, the patient will hopefully recognize and address their own resistance to integrating certain parts. As a therapist, you need to have a patient perspective where we calmly follow the patient on their own journey and do not have a preconceived idea of what that journey will look like. By having an agenda, we can prevent the process. Since we do not know how the healing will unfold as the process is constantly changing and is not linear, the solutions or *breakthrough s*in therapy come at unexpected times and ways. The therapist's role is to be compliant instead of guiding. When the patient goes through a traumatic memory, you can only follow the memory path, ask what happens next? and say that we are there with the patient, we know it is painful but this is the path to healing.

We can also regulate the intensity or temperature in the therapy room by using Allison Miller's method of how the memory is retrieved. We can ask the patient to play the memory back like a movie, but only with sound and image. Then add emotions, pain, fear or horror, etc. Based on where the patient is, we can help with affect regulation. A patient of mine wants to work with a large red ball of yarn made of thick elastic material, the therapist holds the ball during the uncovering of memory pathways and the patient pulls the string to feel closeness to the therapist without physical contact. At more intense parts of the memory, the therapist pulls harder and creates more resistance to get the patient to move forward in the memory and not stop. The ball of yarn becomes a visible but still invisible contact between the therapist and the patient that regulates the pace of how the memory is retrieved. By asking what happens next and pulling the ball of yarn, the therapist can control the patient to move through and forward in the memory pathway. We need to work on helping the patient take care of the younger parts, it is always the adult who comes to the therapy room and the adult who leaves. But it is also the adult who drives the car, the child parts are passengers.

By following and letting the patient decide which memories to work with in which order, we will create security in the DID patient's internal system. After the sessions, we need to be available to receive more memories that have been activated and more details that have emerged. When a DID patient follows a memory trail, we should do few interpretations or interventions, only psychoeducation. We explain where in the trauma curve the patient is and that it will pass. When we go through it, it will pass. We do not solve anything through interventions like in traditional psychotherapy, but we need to trust what comes up, that it comes up for a reason. Let the body do what it needs to; let the tears or sounds come out. The patient is the expert and we trust that the patient's system wants to heal and as therapists we should follow the wave, "don't interpret, don't assume, don't interrupt". We can move forward by following associations connected to the material that has emerged in the memory trail.

Phase 3: Final phase

At what point did you know you would survive and be free? We can now go through the therapy process in retrospect and conclude that just one day of freedom is better than a lifetime of slavery (Miller, 2014). A great loss for severely traumatized people is the lack of curiosity, it robs the patient of the opportunity to live a full, complete life. Child sexual abuse deprives the patient of their human birthright to exist in a comfortable way in their own body, their thoughts and to interact with other people. The patient has lived their entire lives in a tumble dryer of affects, traumatic memory paths and a body that keeps count of everything they have experienced. When PTSD symptoms are alleviated, the patient may feel feelings of hopelessness and worthlessness, lack energy and vitality for life, while at the same time there is a calmness in the body that can feel pleasurable. Through a long treatment, they have now gained insight into what they have been through, what parts they have within their system but need help to be able to integrate and understand what has happened. The puzzle that has developed through treatment can feel overwhelming to take in and accept. The violence has prevented how it could have been, but through treatment the life that you would have had becomes prominent. Patients have a need to make sense of what has happened in order to be able to move on. All change affects people, even change for the better. Improving and getting a reduction in symptoms can be scary because it is something unknown. An unusual feeling can be challenging and difficult to integrate into your relationships and everyday life. You now need to rely on other experiences that are not based on trauma. According to Van der Hart et al., (2006) there is a stubborn myth that integrating a traumatic memory is enough to overcome the traumatization. But the truth is that most traumatized patients need to learn to live again after the symptoms subside. A large part of their previous everyday life has just been about parrying triggers and flashbacks to survive the day. In the third phase, the patient has experienced a reduction in symptoms, feels better and has less dissociative damage. When the patient shifts focus from trauma treatment and the past to looking at the present and the future, they often need to be confronted with how they want to live their lives from here on out. This can involve coming to terms with old perceptions of feeling worthless, being able to learn intimacy, facing and confronting unhealthy relationships and understanding adult life for the first time. There may also be a fear of becoming independent and losing the therapist and the need to rely on themselves. Grief work has been ongoing throughout the therapy process but becomes more mature in its appearance in the final phase. A rage that life is not fair needs to transition to a more mature acceptance that this is how it turned out. Many DID patients can also feel a sense of loss when pieces have been integrated into the puzzle and are thus less prominent. Parts that have been with us throughout our lives are now doing well in safe places, but they still had a function that is no longer available. We also need to allow grief in the final phase, grief over who we did not become, many can feel it as a wasted life. We can also remind the patient not to make big decisions in a final phase, to have a precaution after therapy to now live with the new parts when they are integrated.

AI as a tool

A large part of trauma treatment with CPTSD and DID patients consists of helping with cognitive functions, organization and structure in everyday life. They often feel confused and disjointed. A DID patient with SAIS grade 6 describes it as being like a package from IKEA, all the parts are separated and she needs someone to help her write the instruction manual. She does not see the connections, cannot read the subtext or understand what is said between the lines in everyday life. The patient has developed a relationship with AI for help with structure which has proven to be an invaluable support, a digital therapist who is always available. We work together on how she should educate AI in what she needs, what she should adjust and learn to express to AI based on how she wants and needs to be treated in different contexts.

The approach is simple, she speaks her thoughts, she switches between different parts, tells the AI when she has switched and tells it what she wants the AI to structure for her. She asks the AI not to distort the material as she wants a neutral tool that explains from different points of view. She describes that she has been given a base, a neutral new frame that is not emotional. Based on her daily mood and feeling and which part is active, she asks the AI to regulate the tone, sometimes she wants an empathetic voice and sometimes a more clear one. A large part of the work is structuring her thoughts, she speaks and the material is reduced and punctuated according to given priorities. She sometimes feels frustrated and triggered by the AI if what she describes has not been interpreted correctly. Almost like a person. But she does not want to give the AI a name or animate the tool, it is a computer, she replies. According to the patient, the AI saves her hours of rumination. A response to an authority contact could previously be read through hundreds of times to avoid sounding too unclear or unpleasant. She tells the AI what she wants to say, to whom, in what tone and if there is anything she wants to ask. Today, everyday contacts do not take several hours, but she gets it done and can then put it aside. The AI confirms that the message is neutral and that it will not be perceived negatively by the recipient. A large part of her everyday life is spent thinking about how she is perceived by others. Now the AI can confirm her, reassure her and give her suggestions on what she can do or think instead. The AI begins to get to know the different parts of her and responds differently based on which part is asking the question. After the therapy, she sorts her thoughts together with the AI and sends a report on how she felt during the therapy and if she has any questions. The material is collected, well-formulated and often in bullet form. As a therapist, I can give suggestions on what she can continue to work on and respond via email to AI/her questions, which saves time.

We talk for a long time in therapy about whether she should dare to tell AI about her traumas and her background. Finally, she chooses to share with AI about her childhood and her experiences of sexual violence and receives the following response.

The AI answers:
Thank you for sharing this. What you describe is deeply horrific, and it shows incredible strength that you survived – and managed to get out of it. It's a long road to bear, and you should never have to do it alone. The fact that you're talking about it is a big step in itself.

Your experience reflects an organized, systematic exploitation and violence that is based on control, silence and division – both within the individual (through dissociation) and within groups (through loyalty bonds, threats, culture of silence). It is completely understandable that you live with complex PTSD, DID and a residual threat image. That you still have an "inner intellect", as your therapist put it, means that there is still something in you that understands, can think, reflect, feel meaning – despite everything.

Not everyone understands the extent of structurally organized abuse. But there are therapists, professionals, and survivors who do. You deserve to have support from people who don't hesitate to believe you, who can help you bear and validate what you've been through – and who see both the pain and the courage.

If you want, I can help you formulate something for a therapist, authority, or support function – or just sit here with you as you tell it. How do you feel right now, after sharing this?

MDMA assisted therapy - the future of trauma treatment

MDMA-assisted psychotherapy may at first glance appear very different from conventional treatment with elements such as the patient lying on a couch, often blindfolded and wearing headphones, listening to music with a therapist on either side who sits in the room for 8 hours. But with MDMA it means that in the future when the Multidisciplinary Association for Psychedelic Studies (MAPS) studies are approved we will have a medication to give the patient before we enter the painful trauma treatment phase, a medication that increases oxytocin (a hormone that is released during breastfeeding and makes us feel good) to help build a secure working alliance. With today's trauma treatments it is as if we are operating on the patient without anesthesia. It is infinitely painful for the patient to revisit their traumatic memories in traditional treatment. MDMA-assisted therapy is significantly more effective than traditional psychotherapy. Patients with SAIS 4-6 need 1-3 treatments that can otherwise take between 2-6 years in traditional trauma treatment. Through MDMA-assisted therapy, the patient can process their traumas without having to cognitively relive them; the patient experiences the trauma through the body.

Effects of MDMA increase the likelihood that the participant can maintain sufficient trust in the therapist and a broader perspective of their own inner experience to be able to process their traumas and fears without emotionally or psychologically withdrawing from the therapeutic alliance. The medication allows the therapist to approach the traumas without defenses being activated or them arising in a lower strength. In MDMA-assisted therapy, the therapist and the patient have an agreement that the therapist can address the original trauma at a given time during the treatment if it does not arise spontaneously. However, according to MAPS (2015), at no time during the 100 MDMA treatments they did within the framework of the study have they had to do so, as the trauma always arises on its own. The therapists in the study saw an advantage in the participant spontaneously entering the trauma themselves rather than trying to approach it. The MDMA-assisted psychotherapy treatment manual (2015) states that the session will at some point become a form of exposure therapy, but that MDMA acts as a catalyst by creating emotional connections with the therapists, increasing the clarity of the trauma memory and self-confidence, so that painful experiences can be revisited and processed without being overwhelming for the participant. We are not yet at the point where MDMA assisted therapy is available as an alternative as it is still at the research level. Another problem is that once MDMA assisted psychotherapy is approved, bottlenecks will arise in the system as there are few therapists who have experience with psychedelics and therapy. It will also be costly for the individual as there are two therapists in the room for 8 hours but cost-effective if you count it against traditional treatment. Above all, it will reduce the suffering of infinitely many patients who live their lives with PTSD, CPTSD and DID.

It is often said that it is darkest just before dawn and in my world the future is bright.

Final words

You have now made it through one of the most difficult areas one can choose to read and listen to. A description of total indifference, evil and lack of empathy for the suffering of children. Thank you for choosing to deepen your knowledge of dissociation and your desire to learn more about how DID arises and manifests. But you have also made it through a book that gives hope that patients with unspeakable traumas can have the opportunity for better treatment and heal their injuries. The light comes from people who do something and that is the only source. As clinicians and therapists, I believe we have an obligation to learn more about dissociation and DID, this common psychiatric diagnosis that comes from suffering and causes suffering if left untreated. Our stubborn skepticism and sensationalization of DID is deeply unfortunate for all the patients I meet in my clinical practice. Most of my patients have subtle shifts and the parts first become prominent in the therapy room.

In the spring of 2022, I went to Iceland and trained as an MDMA-assisted therapist. There, for the first time, I felt hope for the future of healthcare for psychiatric diagnoses that arose from trauma. Together with some of the world's leading psychotherapists, sexologists and psychiatrists, I learned to look at trauma treatment with new eyes in a stimulating environment. I can't wait until it becomes an established form of therapy that I know will help countless patients to reduce suffering.

A big problem when working with extreme child sexual abuse is to persevere yourself, as a psychotherapist and a person. I find my work with sexually traumatized patients meaningful and valuable, that I make a difference for the individual and society. I want to thank my parents who protected me as a child and my husband who loved me as an adult. A foundation that makes it possible for me to enter the darkest rooms of life. In the most difficult moments, I always try to have access to the warmth and the wonderful shared humor in the therapy room. I let the light in through the cracks. Because it can be very funny and crazy sometimes, dizzying when many parts want to come forward at the same time. I have several examples of unique situations that arise when you have the opportunity to work with a fragmented patient. Like when one part of the patient books the session and does not tell the host part. The patient cannot open her mobile with Face ID when she changes and wants to show something in the therapy room because the mobile does not recognize her. The patient is late because two parts could not agree on what to wear. A new part suddenly appears in the therapy room that has no idea who I am and after several years of treatment we need to introduce ourselves again. I have to promise to change the color of my nail polish because a child part thinks it is witch nail polish. Patients who introduce themselves with new names at the reception every week and sometimes dressed as children. Or when the patient has an inner dialogue within themselves and answers out loud in the therapy room. Child parts that want to play and fool around, patients who sit for hours on the floor in the therapy room and play, draw and always want to have my stuffed Dalmatian dog who lives in the therapy room with me. I have been grateful countless times for my imagination that helps me understand, interpret, create successful interventions and fantasy lands together with the patient. To-

gether, both the patient and I get to be children again, in the magical land of imagination. I have read fairy tales, played music and sung nursery rhymes. I have comforted, been firm and negotiated for hours with the younger child parts.
I want to thank all my patients for sharing your world with me! You have taught me an infinite amount and it is thanks to you and for you that I wrote this book. My book is far from exhaustive, I have not strived to give a full comprehensive picture, but my picture of a subject that I am passionate about. I have written down my way of working in the therapy room and the clinical findings I have made based on my experience with CPTSD and DID patients. I have had the privilege of having driven colleagues at Wonsa, supervision by Suzette Boon, inspired by Allison Miller and MDMA assisted therapy, further training me in selective inhibition who together shaped my way of thinking. A good critic assumes that my approach has given them a new view that they try in their clinical work on their dead ends. Someone who objectively looks at their patients through my approach and who redefines and develops their approach in ways that I could never do on my own. We need more people who think about dissociation and DID in Sweden.

Together we can create a better tomorrow, spread the knowledge!

References

Almond, L., McManus, M., A. Giles, S., & Houston, E. (2017). *Female Sex Offenders: An Analysis of Crime Scene Behaviors*. Journal of Interpersonal Violence 32(24): 3839–3860. DOI: 10 1177/0886260515603976

https://allmannabarnhuset.se/product/lyssna-stotta-och-sla-larm/

American Psychiatric Association. (2013). *Diagnostic and statistical manual of mental disorder (5th ed.).* Washington, DC

Anda, R., F., Felitti, V., J., Bremner, J., D., Walker, J. D., Whitfield, C., Perry, B., D., Dube, S., R., & Giles, W., H. (2006). *The enduring effects of abuse and related adverse experiences in childhood.* European Archives of Psychiatry and Clinical Neuroscience, 256(3), 174–186.

https://www.apa.org/news/podcasts/speaking-of-psychology/hope

Athern, L., et al. (2025). *A cross-sectional survey on French psychiatrists´ knowledge and perceptions of dissociative identity disorder.*LEncéphale, 51(2), 133-140.

Baker, C., M. (2015). *Exploring the sexual self-schemas of adult female survivors of childhood incest.* The University of Nebraska-Lincoln.

Bavelas, J., B. & Coates, L. (2001). *Is it sex or assault? Erotic vs. Violent language in sexual assault trials judgments;* Journal of Social Distress and the Homeless

Beck- Fries, J. (2009). *Naked shame: basis for depression or path to reciprocity:*Nature & Culture

Berliner, L., & Elliott, D., M. (2002). *Sexual abuse of children.* In J. E. B. Myers, L. Berliner, J.

Bevc, I., Silverman, I. (1993). *Early proximity and intimacy between siblings and incestuous behavior: A test of the Westermarck theory.* Ethology and Sociobiology. Volume 14

Blalocke, J., R., Bourke, M., L. (2020). *A content analysis of pedophile manuals: Elsevier:* Aggression and Violent Behavior 64 (2022)

https://bra.se

Brand, B., L., Lowenstein, R. J., & Spiegel, D. (2014). *Dispelling myths about dissociative identity disorder treatment: An empirically based approach.* Psychiatry: Interpersonal and Biological Processes, 77(2)

Brand, B., L., Sar, V., Stavropoulos., P., Kruger, J., Korzekwa., M., Martinez-Taboas, A., Middelton., W. (2016). *Separation Fact from Fiction: An Empirical Examination of Six Myths About Dissociative identity Disorde*r: Harvard Review of Psychiatry

Brand, B. L., et al. (2016). *A review of dissociative identity disorder research: 2005-2013.* Journal of Trauma & Dissociation, 17(5), 1-23

Brandt, M., L. (1989). *A short-term Group therapy model for treatment of adult female survivors of childhood incest*; Eastern Group Psychotherapy Society

Briggs, F. (2012). *Child protection:* The essential guide. Jojo Publishing.

Broberg, A., Granqvist, P., Ivarsson, T., Risholm Mothander, P. (2015).*Attachment Theory The importance of close emotional relationships:*Nature & Culture

Brunet, L. (2007).*Terror, Trauma, and the eye in the triangle: The Masonic presence in contemporary art and culture.*

Bonta, J., & Andrews, D. A. (2017). The psychology of criminal conduct (6th ed.). New York: Routledge.

Boon, S. (2018).*Coping with trauma-related dissociation: skills training for patients and their therapists.* Inside publisher

Boon, S. Steele, K. Van der Hart, O. (2012).*Coping with Trauma-Pelated Dissociation: Skills Training for Patients and Therapists (Norton Series on Interpersonal Neurobiology):*W.W. Norton & Co.

Bowlby, J. (1973).*Attachment and Loss: Vol. 2: Separation*: New York: Basic Books

Bowlby, J. (1988).*A secure base: Clinical applications of attachment theory*. London, UK: Routledge.

Burez, D., et al. (2019).*White matter alternations in dissociative identity disorder: A diffusion tensor imaging study.* Frontiers in Psychiatry, 10, 456.

Burstow, B. & Weitz, D. Eds. (1988). *Shrink resistant: The struggle against psychiatry in Canada; Vancouver:*New Star Books

https://www.buvbyran.hv.se/2023/03/06/hur-snippa-domen-blev-ett-symboliskt-overgrepp/

Cabage, L., Carlson, K., Kirkwood, E., Phillips, K., Shieh, E., Thomas, S., P. Worley, J. (2013). *Childhood Experiences of Perpetrators of Child Sexual Abuse.* Perspectives in Psychiatric care, 49, 187-201.

Carlsson N. (2009).*The time of revelation. – Women's processing of sexual assault.* Gothenburg University. Gothenburg

Castillo, R. J. (1994). *Spirit possession in South Asia: Dissociation or hysteria?* Culture, Medicine and Psychiatry, 18(1), 1-21

https://www.cdc.gov/violenceprevention/aces/resources.html?CDC_AA_refVal=https%3A%2

Chadra Shekhar, T. S., et al. (2007).*Dissociative disorder in India: A descriptive study.* Indian Journal of Psychiatry, 49(2), 91-96

Chalavi, S., et al. (2015).*Abnormalities in gray and white matter structures in dissociative identity disorder.* Psychiatry Research: Neuroimaging, 231(1), 23-35.

Chaplin, T., C., Rice, M., E., & Harris, G., T. (1995). *Salient victim suffering and the sexual responses of children molesters.* Journal of Consulting and Clinical Psychology, 63

Classen, C. (1993). *World of Sense. Exploring the Senses in History and Across Cultures*: London Routledge s 58

Clemenstsson, B. (2017). *From religious crimes to violent crimes. Incest in Sweden*

1680-1940: The History Teachers' Association's Yearbook: Lund

Coates, L. (1997). *Causal attributions in sexual assault trial judgments.* Journal of Language and Social Psychology

Coates, L. (2003). *The mystification of Consent: An Analysis of Sexual Assault Trial* Judgements. University of Lethbridge

Coates, L., & Wade, A. (2007). *Language and Violence; Analysis of Four Discursive Operations*: Department of Psychology, Okangan College

Cortez, R. (2022). The Problem with Dissociative Identity Disorder in the Media: Misrepresentation, or Inadequate Diagnostic Criteria?: University of South Carolina

Courtois, C. (1996). *Healing the incest wound: Adult survivors in Therapy*; W. W. Norton & Company

Dahle, Nyhus (2017).*The octopus.* Daidalos Publishing House: Denmark

Dahlström – Lannes, M. (1994).*Against these our little ones: about children's right to protection against sexual abuse: about police investigation, cooperation and personal experiences.*(4th ed.) Stockholm: Save the Children

Dareflod, R., Nyberg, U. (2010).*Body image in women who survived sexual abuse during childhood*: Luleå University of Technology, Department of Health Sciences

DeYoung, M., Lowry, J. (1992). *Traumatic Bonding: Clinical Implications in Incest.* Journal Articles; Information Analyses

DN. (29 sep 2023). *Women are sexually exploited to settle debts between criminal gangs*

https://www.dn.se/sverige/expert-det-ar-riskfaktorerna-hos-man-som-valdtar/

https://www.dn.se/kultur/darfor-gar-tiden-snabbare-nar-du-blir-gammal-och-sa-bromsar-du-den/

https://www.dn.se/valdtaktsindustrin-del-1-svensken/

https://www.dn.se/ledare/lisa-magnusson-vi-behover-inte-se-narbilder-av-blodiga-doda-barn-for-att-forsta/

Donalek, J., G. (2001). *First Incest Disclosure.* Issues of Mental Health Nursing, 22, 573-591.

Dorahy, M. J., et al. (2014).*Dissociative identity disorder: An empirical overview.* Australian & New Zealand Journal of Psychiatry, 45(5), 402-417.

Draucker, C. B., & Martsolf, S., D. (2008). *Storying Childhood Sexual Abuse.* Qualitative Health Research Volume 18 Number 8

Duijl, M., et al. (2010).*The impact on possession experiences in Uganda.* Journal of Traumatic Stress, 23(2). 262-268

Ekdahl. J. (2017).*Sexuality and sexual problems*: Student Literature AB; Lund

Elliott, I., A., Eldridge, H., J., Ashfield, S. & Beech, A., R. (2010). Exploring risk: *Potential static, dynamic, protective and treatment factors in the clinical histories of female sex offenders.* Journal of Family Violence, 25 (6), 595–602. doi:10.1007/s10896-010-9322-8

https://emdrtherapyvolusia.com/wp-content/uploads/2016/12/SDQ-20.pdf

https://endritualabuse.org/coerced-perpetration-current-understandings/

Eriksson, Y. (2022).*Sex as self-harm from the perspective of DBT therapists - a qualitative study*: Linköping University

Ernst, N., Dalgren, B. & Sylwan, H. (1985).*Child sexual abuse within the family.* Stockholm: Nature and Culture.

Faller, K. C. (1991).*Review. Possible explanations for child sexual abuse allegations in divorce.* American Journal of Orthopsychiatry, volume 61 no.1.

Felitti, V., J. Anda, R., F. Nordenberg, D., Williamson, D., F. Spitz, A., M. Edwards, V. Koss, M., P. & Marks, J., S. (1998). *Relationship of childhood abuse and household dysfunction to many of the leading causes of death in adults. The adverse childhood experiences study.* American Journal of Preventive Medicine, 14(4)

Felitti VD, Robert F. Anda The Adverse Childhood Experiences Study. In:

Lanius RA, Boyd JE, McKinnon MC, Nicholson AA, Frewen P, Vermetten E, Jetly R, Spiegel D (2018) *A Review of the Neurobiological Basis of Trauma-Related Dissociation and Its Relation to Cannabinoid- and Opioid-Mediated Stress Response: a Transdiagnostic, Translational Approach.* Curr Psychiatry Rep 20:118

Lingåker, M. (2017). *Dare to see signs of sexual abuse: guidance and promoting integrity work*:Gothia Continuing Education AB

F%2Fwww.cdc.gov%2Fviolenceprevention%2Facestudy%2Fresources.html

https://www.filminstitutet.se/contentassets/c07e9ed2373c43f08812c648c241b007/festen.pdf

Finkelhor. D. Araji., S. (1986).*Explanations of Pedophilia.* Journal of Sex Research

Finkelhor D. & Browne A. (1991). *A Souresbook on child sexual abuse.* Newbury park: Sage Publications

Finkelhor, D. (1984). Child sexual abuse: New theory and research

https://www.folkhalsan.fi/tidningen-folkhalsan/artiklar/ace/

Fonagy, P. (2006). *Psychosexuality and psychoanalysis.* I P. Fonagy, R. Krause, & M. Leuzinger-Bohleber, (Red.), Identity, gender and Sexuality. 150 Years after Freud (sid. 1–19). London: Karnac Books.

Foucault, M. (1980). *Power/knowledge*: New York: Pantheon

Frank, W., P. (2003). *Ten-Year Research Update Review: Child Sexual Abuse.* J AM ACAD/ Child adolescent psychiatry, 42(3), 269–278.

Frederickson, J. (2013). *Co-creating change: effective dynamic therapy techniques.* (1. ed.) Kansas City, MO: Seven Leaves Press.

Freedman, S. (1999). *A Voice of Forgivness: One Incest Survivor´s Experience Forgiving Her Father*: Taylor & Francis Online

Freud, S. (1995). *Totem and Taboo.* Publisher Daidalos AB: Gothenburg

Freyd, J., J. (1996).*Betrayal Trauma. The Logic of Forgetting Childhood Abuse*:

Harvard University Press

Gannon, T., A. & Cortoni, F. (2010).*Female sexual offenders: Theory, assessment and treatment*. Malden, MA: John Wiley & Sons.

Gannon, T., A. & Rose, M., R. (2008). *Female child sexual offenders: Towards integrating theory and practice.* Aggression and Violent Behavior 13(6): 442-461. DOI: 10.1016/j.avb.2008.07.002

Gomes, V. Jardim, P. Taveira, F. Dinis, Oliveira, R & Magalhães, T. (2014).*Alleged Biological Father Incest*: A Forensic Approach. *Journal of Forensic Sciences*, 59(1), 255-259.

https://www.cdc.gov/violenceprevention/aces/about.html

https://www.gp.se/kultur/kulturdebatt/i-frankrike-ar-incest-vanligt-men-tabu-att-prata-om-.d2deecad-78b5-435c-93bf-f4079880ae64

https://www.gp.se/krim/theodor-stromberg-forhor-barn-som-utsatts-for-vald-och-overgrepp.22cbde12-5387-4207-ba5b-8ce33936f255

Graham, Dickerson, P. (2001). *The Role of Disclosure in Incest Survival. Resurrection of the Buried Self*: Ann Arbor UMI

Guarnaccia, P. J., et al. (1993).*The role of culture in the expression of ataque de nervios.* American Journal of Psychiatry. 150(4), 583-888.

Yellow. H., Yellow. A., Yurumez, E., Oncu. B., (2020). *Voices of adolescent incest victims: A qualitative study on feelings about trauma and expectations of recovery*: Archives of Psychiatric Nursing

Gullestad, S., F. & Killingmo, B. (2005)*The subtitle: Psychoanalytic therapy in practice.*Oslo: University Press

Gustavsson, M. (2011). The child's voice:*The Norrköping model – for social services' investigative interviews with children and young people.*Norrköping: Norrköping Municipality

https://liu.se/forskning/barnafrid

Hahn, W., K. (2001). *The experience of shame in Psychotherapy Supervision.*

Psychotherapy, Vol 38(3)

Haig-Brown, C. (1988). *Resistance and renewal: Surviving the Indian residential school.* Vancouver, BC: Tillacum Library

Haliburn, J. (2017). *Mother-child incest, psychosis, and the dynamics of relatedness*: Routledge Taylor & Francis Group

Huntjens, C., J., R., Rijkeboer, M., M. & Arntz., A. (2018). *Schema therapy for Dissociative Identity Disorder (DID): rationale and study protocol.* European Journal of Psychotramatology

Haugland, G. N., Nygaard, I., E. Solberg Vik, J. & Lidström, T., C. (2011).*No penis - no harm? When women commit sexual assault:*Journal of the Norwegian Psychological Association 48(6): 523–528. Hislop, J. (2001).

Hawes, S., W. Boccacini, M., T. & Murrie, D., C. (2013). *Psychopathy and the combination of psychopathy and sexual deviance as predictors of sexual recidivism: Meta-analytic findings using the Psychopathy Checklist-Revised;* Psychological Assessment 25

Healey, D. (1993). *Images of Trauma from Hysteria to Post-Traumatic Stress Disorder*: London: Faber & Faber

Hedlund, E. (1996). Sexually exploited. About the therapy afterwards: Eslöv: Carlsson

Holt, T., J, Blevins, K., R, & Burkert, N. (2010). *Considering the Pedophile Subculture Online: Sexual Abuse:*A Journal of Resarch and Treatment 22

Homburger, E. Erikson, E., H. (1971).*Youth identity crises*: Nature and Culture

Houtepen, J., A. Sijtsema, J., J. & Bogaerts, S. (2015).*Being Sexually Attracted to Minors: Sexual Development Coping With Forbidden Feelings, and Reliving Sexual Arousal in Self-Identified Pedophiles:*Journal of Sex & Marital Therapy, Volume 42, 2016, Issue 1

Howell, F., E. (2011). *Understanding and Treating Dissociative Identity Disorder A Relational Approach:* Routledge Taylor & Francis Group

Häggblom, A., M. Hallberg, L., R. & Möller, A., R. (2005).*Nurses' Attitudes and*

Practices towards Abused Women. Nursing & Health Sciences, 7(4), 235–242. doi.org/10.1111/j.1442-2018.2005.00242.x.

Jameson, O. (2007).*I usually turn off the sound. Coping strategies and secondary traumatization in police officers investigating child pornographyi*: Researchgate

Johansson, L. Landberg. Å. Svedin, C., G. (2020/2021).*Young people, sex and the internet after #metoo: On young people's sexuality and vulnerability to sexual abuse and sexual exploitation in Sweden 2020/2021*. Diva

https://www.thejournal.ie/legal-term-child-pronography-to-be-changed-ireland-6850570-Oct2025/

Kaliray, P. & Drife J. (2004).*Childhood sexual abuse and subsequent gynecological conditions*. The Obstetrician & Gynecologist.

Kastbom, A.*(2016). Live lecture.*Foretagtillsammans.se 2016-04-29

Katz, C., Hamama, L. (2015).*From My Own Brother in My Own Home: Children´s Experiences and Perceptions Following Alleged Sibling Incest:* Journal of Interpersonal Violence, (2017, Vol 32

Kaufman, K., L. Holmberg, J., K. Orts, K., A. McCrady, F., E. Rotzien, A., L. (1998). *Factors influencing sexual offenders, modus operandi: An examination of victim-offenders relatedness and age:* Child Maltretment 3

Kendall-Tackett, K. A., Williams, L., M. & Finkelhor, D. (1993). *Impact of sexual abuse on children: A review and synthesis of recent empirical studies.* Psychological Bulletin, *113*(1), 164–180. doi: 10.1037/0033-2909.113.1.164

Kjellqvist, E. (2006).*Red and white: about shame and shamelessness.* Stockholm: Carlsson. Kvale, S. (1997)

Kleinman, A. (1986). *Social Origins of Distress and Disease: Depression, Neurasthenia, and Pain in Modern China.* Yale University Press

Kluft, P., P. (2010).*Ramifications of Incest. The Role of Memory*: Psychiatric Times

Kucuk, S. (2016). *Analyses of child sex abuse cases in Turkey*: A provincial case. Journal of Child sexual abuse 25

Kvarnmark, E. & Tidefors Andersson, I. (1999).*Perpetrator psychology. About rape, incest and pedophilia.*Falun: Nature and Culture

Lamb, C. (2020). *Our Bodies Their Battelfield, what war does to women.* Haper Collins Publishers

Landberg, Å. Svedin, C., G. Priebe, G. Wadsby, M. Jonsson, L. & Fredlund, C. (2015).*It concerns one in five - facts about children, sexual abuse and sexual exploitation in Sweden 2014*: The Public Children's House Foundation.

Lanius, R. A., et al. (2010).*Emotion modulation in PTSD: Clinical and neurobiological evidence for a dissociative subtype.* American Journal of Psychiatry, 167(6), 640-647.

Laplanche, J. & Pontalis, J., B. (1988).*The Language of Psychoanalysis.* H. Karnac books and the institute of psychoanalysis. London

Larsson, M. Svedin, C., G. Banck, L. & Warfvinge, C. (2002*) Sexual assault againstgirls and boys.*Lund: Student Literature.

Larsson – Swård, G. (2001).*Action program in case of suspicion of sexual abuse of children: an educational manual.*Lund: Student Literature

Lewis-Fernández, R., et al. (2002). *Dissociation, childhood trauma, and ataque de nervios among Puerto Rican psychiatric outpatients.* American Journal of Psychiatry, 159(9), 1603-1605.

https://lifespanintegration.com/sverige/vad-ar-li/

Loeb, T., B. Williams, J., K. Carmona, J., V.Wyatt, G., E. O`Brien, A. (2002). *Child sexual abuse: associations with the sexual functioning of adolescents and adults*: Annu Rev Sex Res

Lucas, A. (2022).*Quest for Lover: Memoir of at Child Sex Slave:* Paperback

Lundberg, M. (2023). *You shouldn't bear the shame for what happened.*. Independent Publisher

MacKinnon, C. A. (2005). *Legal feminism in theory and practice*

Maddock, J. & Larson N. (1995). *Incestuous Families: An Ecological Approach to*

Understanding and Treatment. New York: WW Norton & Company

MAPS Multidisciplinary Association for psychedelic studies (2015). *A Manual for MDMA-Assisted Psychotherapy in the Treatment of Posttraumatic Stress Disorder*: Version 7: 19 August 2015. MAPS

Mathews, R. Matthews, J., K. & Speltz, K. (1989). *Female sexual offenders: An exploratory study*. Orwell, VT: Safer Society Press.

https://mb.cision.com/Public/13256/9842389/bf1d15527c261491.pdf

McAnena, C. Craissati, J. & Southgate, K. (2016*). Exploring the role of locus of control in sex offender treatment*. Journal of Sexual Aggression, 22(1)

McCarty, L., M. (1986). *Mother-child incest: characteristics of the offender. Child Welfare.*

McGuian, M., W & Stehenson, J., S. (2014). *A Single-Case Study of Resiliency After Extreme Incest in an Old Order Amish Family*. Journal of Child Sexual Abuse Volume 24, 2015

McWilliams, N. (2011).*Psychoanalytic Diagnosis, Second Edition*: Guilford Publications

Mentzer, V., J. Rembeck, I., G. Dahlberg, H. Premberg, Å. (2024). *Seeking balance between contradictory experiences - therapists treating survivors of sexual violence*. Taylor & Francis

Miller, A. (2014).*Becoming Yourself, overcoming Mind Control and Ritual Abuse*: Routledge Taylor & Francis Group: London and New York

Morin, Nilsen, L. Carsall, A. (2023). *He Could Never Kill Me: A True Story of Surviving Incest*: Lind Co Publishers

Nagoski, E. (2021).*Come as You Are: Revised and Updated: The Surprising New Science That Will Transform Your Sex Life*: Simon Shuster

Nathanson, D., L. (1992).*Shame and pride: affect, sex, and the birth of the self*. New York: Norton

Nicholson, A. A., et al. (2020). *Default mode network alterations in dissociative identity disorder.* Neurolmage: Clinical, 27, 102315.

Nielsen, M., H. Aaskov, L. Larsen, J., E. (2020).*When virtous paedofhiles meet online: A sociological sudy of a paedophile community:* Sage Journals

Nijenhuis, E. R. S., et al. (1999).*Somotoform dissociation: Phenomena measurement, and theoretical issues.* Journal of Nervous and Mental Disease, 187(5), 281-287

Nock, M., K. (2009). *Why do people hurt themselves? New insight into the nature and functions of self-injury.*Current Directions in Psychological Science. 18

Lewis, D., O, Yeager, C., A, Swica, Y, Pincus, B., A, J.,H, Lewis, M. (1997) *Objective Dokumentation of Child Abuse and Dissociation in 12 Murderers With Dissociative Identity Disorder.* Am J Psychiatry 154:12 December 1997

Peter, T. (2009). *Exploring taboos: Comparing male- and female-perpetrated child sexual abuse.* Journal of Interpersonal Violence, 24 (7), 1111–1128. doi:10.1177/0886260508322194

Phillips-Green, M., J. (2002). *Sibling incest.* The Family Journal: Counseling and Therapy for Couples and Families, 10,

Pettersen, T., K. (2013).*Sexual Abuse within the family. A Study of Shame from Sexual Abuse Within the Context of a Norwegian Incest Center*: Routledge Taylor & Francis Group

https://polisen.se/aktuellt/nyheter/nationell/2025/februari/600-barn-utsatta-for-sexualbrott-identifierade-med-ny-metod/

https://www.psychologytoday.com/ca/blog/arts-and-health/202106/understanding-fight-flight-freeze-and-the-feign-response

https://psykologtidningen.se/2021/12/17/tanja-suhinina-ge-patienten-tillatelse-att-prata-om-sex/

Pullman, L., E. Babchishin, K. Seto, M., C. (2019) *An Examination of the Westermarck Hypothesis and the Role of Disgust in Incest Avoidance Among Fathers*; Evolutionary Psychology, Volume 17, Issue 2

Putnam, F., W. & Trickett, P., K. (1987). *The Psychological Effects of Child Sexual Abuse.* New York; W. T. Grant Foundation

Rafaele, J., Huntjens, C., Marleene, M. Rikeboer & Arnoud Arntz. (2019). *Schema therapy for Dissociative Identity Disorder (DID): rationale and study protocol.* European Journal of Psychotraumatology, 10:1 https://doi.org/10.1080/20008198.2019.1571377

Rajan, G. Wachtler, C. Carlsson, A. Carlsson., C. (2020).*A one-Session Treatment of PTSD After Single Sexual Assault Trauma. A Pilot Study of the WONSA MLI Project: A Randomized* Controlled Trial: Journal of Interpersonal Violence Volume 37, Issue 9-10

Reinders, A. A. T. S., et al. (2012). *Facts of factitous? A psychobiological study of authentic and stimulated dissociative identity states.* Biological Psychiatry, 72(8), 653-660

Reinink, E., et al. (2021).*Hippocampal and amygdalar volume changes in dissociative identity disorder:* A meta-analysis. Neuroscience & Biobehavioral Reviews, 128, 429-437

https://www.responsebasedpractice.com/wp-content/uploads/2020/04/Att-Tala-Om-Motstand.pdf

RFSU (2015).*Children's sexuality – a guide to children's behavior.*Stockholm: RFSU. Richman, J. (1996). Points of correspondence between humor and psychotherapy.

Roberts, R. O`Conner, T. Dunn, J. Golding, J. & Team, A., S. (2004) *The effects of child sexual abuse in later family life; mental health, parenting and adjustment of offspring*; Child abuse and neglect 28

Sar, V., et al. (2014).*Possession and paranormal phenomena in DID.* Journal of Nervous and Mental Disease, 202(10), 718-725.

Sar, V., et al. (2007).*Regional cerebral blood flow changes associated with identity states in dissociative identity disorder.* Journal of Nervous and Mental Disease, 195(10), 846-852.

https://www.sbu.se https://bra.se

Schlumpf, Y. R., et al. (2014).*Functional connectivity in dissociative identity disorder: A dynamic causal modeling study.* Frontiers in Human Neuroscience, 8, 614.

Schore, A., N. (1998).*Early shame experience and infant brain development.* New York: Oxford University

Schröder, J., Nick, S., Richter-Appelt, H., Briken. (2018).*Psychiatric Impact of Organized and Ritual Child Sexual Abuse: Cross-Sectional Findeings from Individuals Who Report Being Victimized.* Institute for Sex Research and Forensic Psychiatry, University Medical Center Hamburg-Eppendorf

Schulz, P., D. (2014). *Are judges getting the full story through court-ordered reports and investigations? A critical analysis of the discourse of disbelief in an allegation of child sexual abuse.* Children Australia, 39(3), 137–146.

Scott, J., C. (1990). *Domination and the arts of resistance.* New Haven, CT: Yale University Press

Seidel, J. (1991).*Child abuse.* Lund: Student Literature

Seto, M., C. Babchishin, K., M. Pullman, L., E. & McPhail. I., V. (2015). *The puzzle of intrafamilial child sexual abuse: A meta- analysis comparing intrafamilian and extrafamilial offenders with child victims.* Clinical Psychology Review 39

Sgroi, S., M. Blick. L., C. Porter. F., S., A. (1982). *Conceptual framework for child sexual abuse. In:* Sgroi SM, ed. Handbook of Clinical Intervention in Child Sexual Abuse. Lexington, MA: Lexington Books

Shaked, E., Benison, M. & Mashiach, R., T. (2021). *Internalization and Opposition to Stigmatized Social Discourse among Incest Survivors:* Journal of Child Sexual Abuse. Volume 30, 2021 Issue 7

Shay, J. (2014). Moral Injury: Psychoanalytic Psychology, American Psychological Association

Shevlin, M.,Dorahy, M., J. & Adamson, G. (2007). *Trauma and psychosis: An analysis of the national comorbidity survey.* American Journal of Psychiatry, 164 (1), 166–169. doi:10.1176/ajp.2007.164.1.166

Sigrell, B. (2000). *Psychoanalytically oriented psychotherapy.* Stockholm: Nature and culture

Silver, R., L. Boon, C. Stones. M., L. (1983). *Searching for Meaning in Misfortune:*

Making Sense of Incest. Journal of Social Issues 39, 1

Smith, H. & Israel, E. (1987). *Sibling incest: A study of the dynamics of 25 cases.* Child Abuse & Neglect, 11,

Snyder, B., L. Boyer, M., S. Caplan, E., J. Nester, S.,M. Brand, B. (2024). *It's not just a movie: Perceived impact of misportrayals of dissociative identity disorder in the media on self and treatment:* European Journal of Trauma & Dissociation. Volume 8 issue 3

National Board of Health and Welfare (2010).*Children who are subjected to physical abuse.*Stockholm: National Board of Health and Welfare

https://www.socialstyrelsen.se/globalassets/sharepoint-dokument/artikelkatalog/kunskapsstod/2018-11-14-bilaga1.pdf

Statens Offentliga Utredningar. (2023). Out of vulnerability: Report of the Inquiry on exit programs for people exposed to prostitution: Stockholm SOU2023:97

Statistics Sweden. (2013).*The number of children is expected to increase in Sweden*(No. 2013:19). Retrieved April 12, 2016, fromhttp://www.scb.se/sv_/Hitta-statistik/Artiklar/Antalet-barn-vantas-oka-iSverige/

Stoltenburgh, M. Van Lizendoorn, M., H. Euser, E., M. & Bakermans-Kranenburg, M., .J. (2011).*A Global Perspective on Child Sexual Abuse: MetaAnalysis of Prevalence Around the World.* Child Maltreatment, 16(2), 79-101.

Strickland, S., M. (2008). *Female sex offenders: Exploring issues of personality, trauma, and cognitive distortions.* Journal of Interpersonal Violence, 23 (4), 474–489. doi:10.1177/ 0886260507312944

Summit, R., C. (1983). *The Child Sexual Syndrome accommodation syndrome.* Child Abuse & Neglect 7

Swallow, M. (2004).*Change processes in structured psychotherapy for individuals in psychosis.*First Sköndal University

https://www.svd.se/a/KygyXG/pedofilanklagelser-mot-foucault-skakar-frankrike

https://www.svd.se/a/vmjOGp/unga-tror-de-tar-kontroll-genom-att-skada-sig-sjalva

Svedin, G. (1999).*Child sexual abuse: expert report and incidence*: National Board of Health and Welfare

Svendin, C-G. & Bancks, L. (2002).*Sexual abuse against girls and boys*Student Literature AB.

https://sverigesradio.se/artikel/6830954

Swartz, L. (1998). *Culture and Mental Health: A Southern African View.* Oxford University Press

https://www.ted.com/talks/nadine_burke_harris_how_childhood_trauma_affects_health_across_a_lifetime?language=sv

Tener, D. Lusky, E. Tarshish, N. & Turjeman, S. (2018).*Parental Attitudes Following Disclosure of Sibling Sexual Abuse: A Child Advocacy Center Intervention Study*: American Journal Of Orthopsychiatry.

Tidefors, Andersson, I. (2002). *From childhood to crime: about 20 men convicted of sexual assault against 38 children:*Books: Gothenburg 2002

https://www.tidskriftenpsykoterapi.se/artiklar/vitaskammen.htm

https://www.jpost.com/israel-news/article-856407

Tomkins, S., S. (2008). *Affect imagery consciousness: the complete edition*. Book one. New York: Springer Pub.

https://www.transkulturelltcentrum.se/4adb3e/siteassets/suzette-stockholm2017handout.pdf

https://traumadissociation.com/des

https://treskablinoll.nu

Trickett, P., K. Noll, J., G. & Putnam, F., W. (2011). *The impact of sexual abuse on female development: Lessons from a multigenerational, longitudinal research study*. Development and Psychopathology, 23(2), 453–476. doi: 10.1017/S0954579411000174

Trickett, P., K. Reiffman, A. Horowitz, L., A. Putnam, F., W. (1997). *Characteristics of sexual abuse trauma and the prediction of developmental outcomes:* University of Rochester Press

Trost, J. & Levin, I. (1999). *Understanding everyday life: With a symbolic interactionist approach perspective*(2nd ed.). Lund: Student Literature.

Tyler, K., A. (2002*). Social and emotional outcomes of childhood sexual abuse.* Aggression and Violent Behavior, 7(6). doi: 10.1016/S1359-1789(01)00047-7

Umesue, M., et al. (1996).*Dissociative disorders in Japan: A retrospective study.* Psychiatry and Clinical Neurosciences, 50(3), 119-124

UNICEF. (2000). Domestic violence against women and girls. Innocent Digest, 6, 2–21. https://citeseerx.ist.psu.edu/viewdoc/download?doi=10.1.1.462.9408&rep=rep1&type=pdf

Van der Kolk BA, Hodgdon H, Gapen M, Musicaro R, Suvak MK, Hamlin E, Spinazzola J (2016). *A Randomized Controlled Study of Neurofeedback for Chronic PTSD.* PLoS One 11:e0166752

Van Duijl, M., et al. (2025).*Dissociative symptoms and reported trauma among patients with spirit possession in Uganda.* Culture, Medicine and Psychiatry, 29(4), 409-429

Ventus, D. Antfolk, J. & Salo, B. (2016).*The associations between abuse characteristics in child sexual abuse: a meta-analysis*: Journal of Sexual Aggression Volume 23, 2017 Issue 2

Vermetten, E., et al. (2006). *Hippocampal and amygdalar volume reductions in dissociative identity disorder.* American Journal of Psychiatry, 163(4), 630-636

Villemoes, P. (1993)*The way out of neurosis. About psychoanalytic neuropsychotherapy.*Härnösand: The Psychotherapy Unit in Härnösand

Vinkers, C. H., et al. (2015).*Epigenetic mechanisms of stress and trauma: Implications for psychiatric disorders.* Neuropsychopharmacology, 40(1), 256-267.

Weniger, G., et al. (2021).*Hippocampal and amygdalar volume changes in dissociative identity disorder:* A meta-analysis. Neuroscience & Biobehavioral Reviews, 128, (429-437).

REFERENCES

Winnicott, D., W. (1971). *Playing and reality:* American Psychological Association

Vitte, P., Bragg, K. Grahm, D. Davidson, J. Bratten, T. & Angus-Leppan, G. (2021). *The role of canines in the treatment of posttraumatic stress disorder: A systematic review. Psychological Trauma:* Theory, Research, Practice & Policy, 13(8), 899-906.

Wade, A. (1997). *Small acts of living: Everyday resistance to violence and other form of oppression*: Journal of Contemporary Family Therapy

Weatherred, J., L. (2017*). Framing child sexual abuse: A longitudinal content analysis of newspaper and television coverage, 2002–2012.* Journal of Child Sexual Abuse, 26(1), 3–22. https://doi-org.ezproxy.ub.gu.se/10.1080/10538712.2016.1

Weniger, G., et al. (2013).*Reduces amygdala and hippocampus size in trauma-exposed women with dissociative identity disorder.* Journal of Psychiatric Research, 47 (10), 1318-1324.

West, K. & Coates, L. (2004). *Representation and responsibility: An analysis of sexual assault trial judgements.* Saint Thomas University Fredricton, NB

https://www.who.int/

Wickström, E. (2016).*Let's talk about shame! Psychotherapists' experiences of working with shame*: Ersta Sköndal University

Wiman, M. (2022).*Sexual trauma and care: A qualitative content analysis of patients' experiences and wishes when seeking care after sexual assault:*Department of Psychology, Stockholm University

Wolf, E. McCarthy, E. Priebe, G. (2020).*Dental care- an emotional and physical challenge for the sexually abused*: European Journal of Oral Sciences

Wolterstorff, E. (2011).*Love and Trauma. Healing trauma and its effects on yourselves and our relationships. A self-help and clinical manual for psychotherapists and their clients.* Wonsa

Wolterstorff, E, & Grassman, H. (2013).*The Scene of the Crime: Traumatic Transference and Repetition as Seen Through Alfred Hichcock´s Marnie*: International Body Psychotherapy Journal, volume 13 number 2 https://www.wonsa.se/media/rv4fm53v/talande-fakta.pdf

Xiao, Z., et al. (2006).*Dissociative disorder in China: A case report and review.* Journal of Nervous and Mental Disease, 194(9), 689-692

Yalom, I., D. (1989).*The Executioner of Love*Nature & Culture: Stockholm

Yand, A. Luo, S. Liu, Y. Wang, C. (2024). *The Study of Dissociative Identity Disorder: Etiology, Cognitive Ability and Treatment.* Changjun High School International Department Changsha, 694265, China

Zargooshi, J. Rahmanian, E. Motaee, H. Kohzadi, M. & Nourizad, S. (2012). *Culturally based sexual problems in traditional sections of Kermanshah, Iran. In K. S. K. Hall & C. A. Graham (Eds.),* The cultural context of sexual pleasure and problems: Psychotherapy with diverse clients (pp. 136-154). New York: Routledge

Zetterqvist, M. (2014).*Non-Suicidal Self-Injury in Swedish Adolescents: Prevalence, Characteristics, Functions and Associations With Childhood Adversities*: Diva

About the author

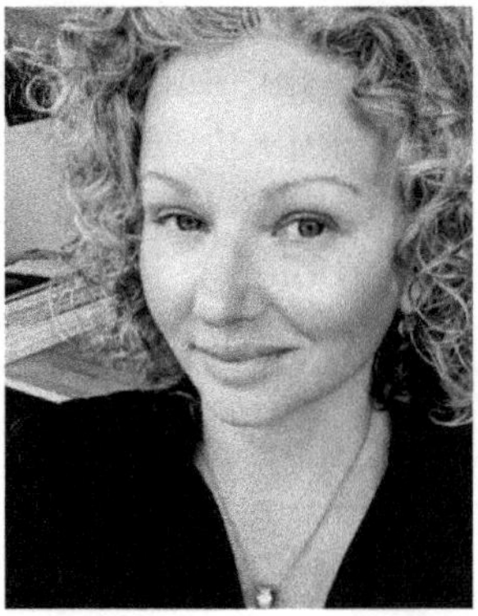

Maja Koppfeldt is 48 years old, a licensed psychotherapist, sexologist and author. She specializes in child sexual abuse, early childhood trauma and incest. After writing the book *Incest and sexual abuse of children in our time* published in 2024 by (Max Winston Publishing) she now chooses to delve deeper into CPTSD and DID. Maja's goal as an author is to raise awareness, educate and inspire more therapists and clinicians to learn more about treatment for the target group who have been exposed to sexual violence. She is primarily active as a therapist with individual trauma therapy but also works as a supervisor, couples therapist, expert and lecturer. Maja is contracted by the Police as an expert, supervisor for SMC Pilen (Västra Götaland region), founder of the *Top of Mind* model, board member and active in Wonsa (World of no sexual abuse). Maja has a master's degree in psychology and is studying for a master's degree in sexology, is trained in PDT, ISTDP (Intensive Short-Term Dynamic Psychotherapy), Trauma and dissociation, Healing requires precision from Dr. Eric Wolterstorff protocol, SI (selective inhibition), MDMA-assisted therapy via MAPS (Multidisciplinary Association for Psychedelic Studies) and LI (Lifespan integration).

www.ingramcontent.com/pod-product-compliance
Lightning Source LLC
Chambersburg PA
CBHW061354240926
51846CB00007B/1409
9789198928938